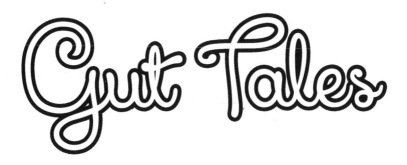

EMMA BECKER

Copyright © 2017 Emma Becker

The content of this book is for general instruction only. Each person's physical, emotional, and spiritual condition is unique. The instruction in this book is not intended to replace or interrupt the reader's relationship with a physician or other professional. Please consult your doctor for matters pertaining to your specific health and diet. Information in this book is general and is offered with no guarantees on the part of the author or publisher. The authors and publisher disclaim all liability in connection with the use of this book.

To contact the author, visit Website: www.HauteWellness.com

ISBN-10: 0-9982710-1-2

ISBN-13: 978-0-9982710-1-9

Printed in the United States of America

Library of Congress Control Number: 2017944926

Promoting Natural Health, LLC, Fort Mill, SC

Dedication

To Dr. Martin L. Greene, M.D.

I am forever indebted to you for saving not only my life, but my colon. I will never forget the care and dedication you showed me when I was at the sickest I have ever been. I will forever carry you in my heart.

To Dr. Brindusa Truta, M.A.S., M.D.

Thank you for going above and beyond to ensure I stayed healthy while pregnant. I am forever appreciative of your dedication and care. My little boy is strong and healthy today because of your guidance, passion, and wisdom. I am forever grateful to you.

To my husband, Matt.

Thank you for holding me up during the darkest, sickest moments of my life. Your love and compassion has been the ongoing antidote I need to not only manage Inflammatory Bowel Disease, but to thrive and live as normal a life as I can. I also thank you for stepping back and allowing me to fully experiment on myself, and gently redirecting me when needed, through my quest to find something that would "cure" me. Though an unknown amount of time, energy, and resources has been spent on researching and carrying out various wellness trends, the best remedy to calm my colon has been right next to me the entire time—you. I love you, Mi Amor.

Table of Contents

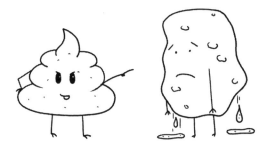

Introduction

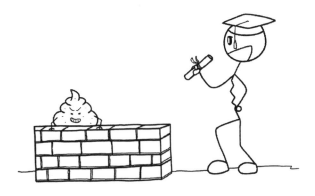

There I was, sitting on top of the world, feeling invincible. I was twenty-four years old, had graduated from one of the best colleges in the nation a year prior, had a fantastic job as an Intelligence Officer, and was blessed with a young, handsome stud of a husband. I felt like I could rule the world and that nothing was going to stop me! I felt that my future was bright and that health and success was promised. I felt so happy-go-lucky as everything had always gone the way I planned. That is, until I found myself young, fabulous, and sick. Wait, what?! Sick?!! Uncontrollable bowel movements? No way! Bloody poo? Say, bloody who?! A chronic disease? What does that *even* mean?

Ladies and gents, it means that my young, fabulous self was diagnosed with severe ulcerative colitis. This also meant, unbeknownst to me, that I was going to have little-to-no control of the tiny fun-sucker muscle named the sphincter. I also had absolutely no idea that my life was going to revolve around poop, doctors' offices, infusion centers, more poop, medication monstrosities, and total breakdowns.

While sitting on the toilet, doubled over in pain and having exploding bloody diarrhea coming out of my arse, I wondered why the hell there were no books on the market explaining what the disease is *really* like. I was over the scientific explanation type books. Finding out the exact scientific definitions, reasoning, and side effects of treatments and disease activity wasn't what I really needed at the time. I needed the raw, real, and dirty details about what to expect with inflammatory bowel disease so there would be no surprises! I would have totally appreciated a heads up from somebody that one day I would be crapping into a paper grocery bag in the back of my car!

That is when the idea for this book was born. In the following pages, I hold nothing back. The lowdown on diets tried, poop accidents had, tears shed, and life changing moments are all documented in the pages to come.

Whether you are newly diagnosed or have struggled with Crohn's disease or ulcerative colitis for years, I'm here to tell you that you are much stronger than your sphincter! You can, and will, get through the tough times of the disease. It's a big kick in the pants, or…colon, to receive such a diagnosis, but I assure you, if looked at through the right frame of mind, it is manageable. You might even be able to kick it out of your life for years.

So, grab a glass of your favorite beverage, clench your sphincter, and let's embark on this ass-kicking journey together!

Ignorance Is Not Bliss

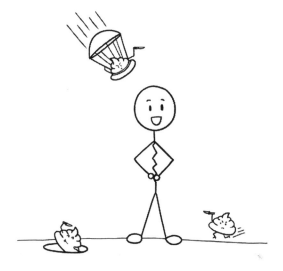

If you are reading this book, odds are you have been diagnosed, or know somebody who has been diagnosed, with Crohn's disease or ulcerative colitis. Crohn's disease and ulcerative colitis are known as inflammatory bowel disease or IBD. NO, this is NOT the same as irritable bowel syndrome. Those assholes, quite literally, get off a bit easier than your asshole, my friend. In short, IBD is shit with a much more serious attitude; not just a case of "OMG, I'm going to shit my pants…find me a bathroom NOW!"

Crohn's and colitis are known by the scientific and medical community as chronic diseases that wax and wane, or come and go, throughout one's lifetime once diagnosed. Because the symptoms are relatively similar for Crohn's and colitis, let's dig into the dirty details of what to expect when you go into a "flare," a.k.a. get sick with symptoms. The not-so-pleasant symptoms of IBD include anal bleeding, bloody poo, severe cramping, blood loss, and the need to be near a bathroom when sick—NONE of which I knew when I was newly diagnosed.

Crohn's disease can affect the entire digestive tract, from the mouth to the anus, though it most commonly affects the end of the small intestine (the ileum) and the beginning of the large intestine. Ulcerative colitis affects the large intestine or colon. Both diseases cause inflammation and potential damage to the bowel, depending on the severity. Keep in mind that, for example, though two individual people have been diagnosed with Crohn's disease, they can have entirely different symptoms and severities of the disease. Now that I've given you an overview of the disease, let me tell you about the discovery of my sick colon.

One spring morning, with birds chirping outside of my bathroom window, I was taking my daily dump when I happened to turn around, look into the toilet, and see bloody poo starring back at me. "AAAHHH! What the hell is that?!!" I then proceeded to do what any normal, rational person would do. I ignored it! I was certain it was a hiccup and would go away on its own. After a week of Count Dracula style poo continuously showing up in my toilet, I decided I better see my primary care doctor "just in case."

I saw my primary care doc the following morning only to be told that they wanted a few small stool samples to ensure it was actually blood that I had in my stool. Being young and dumb, I was a bit frustrated because red beets weren't a normal part of my diet, so what the hell else would be causing my poo to be red in appearance?! *Let's get real doc, quit wasting my time!* I thought.

After the results of the stool sample came back and tested positive for blood, I was referred to a gastroenterologist. I wasn't sure what the heck a gastroenterologist was but went only because I was still bleeding out of my bum and was starting to feel a bit run down and weak.

After the first few minutes of my appointment with a gastroenterologist, I figured out pretty quickly that this particular doc was a subject matter expert in all things poop and wanted to know, quite literally, all the dirty details about my daily bowel movements!! I was a bit entertained during the first appointment as I had never focused solely on my asshole, my poop, the smell of my poop or the color, consistency, or frequency of my poop!

During my initial appointment, the gastroenterologist decided that the only way to truly figure out what was causing the bloody diarrhea was to conduct a colonoscopy. I was scheduled for a colonoscopy a month later and went about my day. At the age of twenty-four, I couldn't quite wrap my mind around the importance of a colonoscopy nor the severity of my situation.

At the time, I wasn't alarmed that my colonoscopy was scheduled for a month out because, naturally, I didn't think my situation was as dire as it truly was. The only aspect of the colonoscopy I was concerned about was the fact that I would have to go on a clear liquid diet the day before and drink a big freaking jug of a mystery solution called "GoLYTELY" so I could clear out my colon to prepare for the colonoscopy.

As I was awaiting my colonoscopy appointment, I found my bloody diarrhea getting more frequent, the lower abdominal cramping getting more severe, and my body becoming weaker and weaker. At the two-and-a-half week mark, I was fifteen pounds lighter and looked like a skeleton covered in pale skin due to crapping high amounts of blood and poo. Though I was crapping blood, losing weight and feeling weaker, I still didn't believe I was *that* sick. It wasn't until meeting a group of friends at our favorite local Mexican joint and indulging in queso dip, a huge chicken burrito covered in more queso, lots of chips and salsa, and a frozen strawberry margarita that reality set in.

About fifteen minutes after leaving the Mexican restaurant, I began experiencing intense cramping that, for the first time, caused me to double over in pain. I slowly made my way to the bathroom, sat my bum down on the toilet, and immediately felt warm blood coming out of my arse. There was no poo, no diarrhea, just warm blood leaking out of my ass. To say I was a bit concerned is an understatement. I ended up spending close to forty-five minutes on the commode with on and off cramping. When my lower abdominals would cramp, it was a precursor that warm blood was on its way out. When all was said and done, I looked into the toilet, and in much horror, saw a toilet bowl full of nothing but blood.

The next morning, I called the gastroenterologist's office and asked if they had any cancellations for colonoscopies as I felt I needed to get in ASAP. The receptionist politely said, "I'm sorry, we do not. You're going to have to wait another week and a half."

"I'm not going to make it that long." I replied in desperation, truly believing that I might meet my untimely demise if they didn't schedule me earlier. She briefly put me on hold before coming back thirty seconds later, telling me she would schedule me for the following week. Though I wasn't looking forward to the colonoscopy prep, I was looking forward to finding out what the heck was going on with my body.

The day of my colonoscopy prep, I wasn't too happy about being on a liquid diet, and I was definitely not looking forward to drinking the mysterious four liter "GoLYTELY" jug. Trying to make it as painless as possible, I filled the massive jug up with water that morning and put it in the fridge so it would be nice and cool by evening. I continued to drink water and chicken broth throughout the day. I was unwilling to eat the "allowed" liquid foods such as Jell-O and popsicles because I wanted to make sure my colon was empty! In my mind, I thought this procedure was only going to happen to me once in my young life and I wanted to do it right!

Around 5pm, I broke out the cold jug of GoLYTELY and took my first eight ounces down like a champ. Ten minutes later, I drank another eight ounces and thought that perhaps this experience wouldn't be too bad. My tummy hadn't started gurgling, and other than feeling hungry, I felt pretty normal. If anything, I thought I was just getting extra hydrated. I soon learned I couldn't have been more wrong!

An hour down and forty-eight ounces later, my asshole started quivering and I rushed to the bathroom. What commenced should never be put onto paper, but for the purposes of this book, I'll make an exception. My asshole exploded like a freaking nuclear bomb once I put my bum on the commode! If it weren't for the containment of the toilet bowl, shit would have gotten everywhere! The velocity of this flying shit was out of this world.

And then it hit me! The benign looking jug, because of its name, GoLYTELY, tricked me into thinking it wouldn't produce such powerful and frequent 'rhea! I think a more accurate name would be GoEXPLODING or GoNUCLEAR because that is exactly what happened to me for the next several hours! The disheartening part of this entire colonoscopy "prep" experience was that blood accompanied each and every explosion, but again, it wasn't necessarily a surprise.

Alas, I finished the jug, exploded some more, and called it a night! At that moment, I knew I would never, ever forget that GoLYTELY was named to trick me, and others, into thinking it would provide a pleasant pooping experience! Great marketing, but not so great in accurately capturing the picture of what would happen to your asshole and your commode!

I awoke the morning of the colonoscopy, ready to get this thing done and to find out what was wreaking havoc on my gut. Once I was wheeled into the surgery room, I totally passed out due to the anesthesia. I just remember groggily waking up to my gastroenterologist. His face pretty much told me all I needed to know, but I still asked, "It was bad, wasn't it?"

"Yes, pretty bad. Your entire colon was ulcerated," he replied. It was at that moment that I was diagnosed with ulcerative colitis, though I was completely oblivious to what that actually meant.

After making a follow-up appointment, I was sent on my way with a shiny bottle of prednisone, screen shots of my severely ulcerated colon, and the world again at my feet. Within a few days of taking prednisone, my symptoms completely disappeared. I truly thought ulcerative colitis was a one-time incident; a sickness I somehow picked up and had now gotten over. I was fixed! Cured! Healed! Unfortunately, I couldn't have been more wrong.

After my colonoscopy, the gastroenterologist failed to tell me that ulcerative colitis was a "chronic illness" and was not the same as having a cold or the flu. Heck, I thought my colon caught the flu, was fixed with prednisone and all better! Who knows, maybe he didn't want to burst my bubble, but damn, it would have helped to know! Looking back, I completely acknowledge that there is no guarantee that I would have understood or accepted what a diagnosis of ulcerative colitis actually meant.

About a month after tapering off prednisone, ulcerations decided to yet again overtake my colon, causing extreme cramping, weight loss, and a bloody poo party in my toilet. When I experienced symptoms for a second time, or a "relapse" of the disease, I decided to order any and all books that pertained to inflammatory bowel disease. Whether the books were scientific or dietary, I read them all. I was hungry for knowledge because I wanted to know exactly what was happening to me and how I could fix it! It wasn't until I read about ulcerative colitis and Crohn's disease in scientific literature that I finally realized the magnitude of the beast living in my gut. It was also then that I realized that the vicious "flare" cycle had begun for me. What I didn't know was how this flare cycle was going to rock my world, and not in a good way.

The best thing I could have done for myself was to read as many books about ulcerative colitis and Crohn's disease that I could get my hands on. In a way, this helped me become my own advocate. Having my colonoscopy pictures helped give me a visual of the ulcer show going on in my gut. They decided to have an entire block party, and my poor colon was the life of the party. For the life of me, I couldn't figure out how these teeny-tiny ulcers were causing so much pain and dysfunction in my life, but the books helped put it into perspective—though it was a perspective I did not want to accept. What was hardest for me to accept was the various drugs that I would have to take during my struggle to remain in remission. The books and scientific literature that broke down medications and potential side effects were, to me, grim at best. I naturally thought I wouldn't need the potent drugs, but life had a funny way of showing me that I had no clue what medications I did and did not need.

The best advice I can give is to become your own advocate, and in doing so, do as much research as possible about your individual disease. If you're not sure what your digestive tract or colon looks like then Google that shit. There are plenty of unedited ulcerated colon and sick digestive tract pictures all over the internet! Had I not read as many books as I could get my hands on, I have no idea when I would've figured out that ulcerative colitis simply wasn't going to go away on its own. I had to undergo a massive lifestyle change; one you will read about in the following chapters. When it comes to IBD, ignorance is NOT bliss! Do your research, trust your instincts, put your "hope" hat on, know that controllable poo is possible, and believe that you can heal!

███ ██ ████ / █ █ ████ ▐██ ▌▟ ████ / █ ████ ██ ██ ▐██ ▌▟ █

At twenty-four years old, I never questioned what drugs were being prescribed for my condition. I just hoped to God they would put me in remission and that I would stop crapping bloody poo fifteen to twenty times a day when flaring. I ran up the drug pyramid pretty quickly and experienced unique side effects, both mentally and physically, to prove it. It took several years for me to realize the magnitude of the drugs coursing through my veins.

As I mentioned, I was first put on prednisone, but I was also put on Lialda immediately after being diagnosed. I experienced rage, hair loss, rashes on my stomach, neck, arms and legs, weight gain (a.k.a. the *marshmallow man syndrome*), night sweats, insomnia, paranoia, and anxiety from the 'roids. Prednisone would put my body into remission pretty quickly, but within a month of tapering off, I would start to flare again. After a year of this brutal tapering dog and pony show, my gastroenterologist decided to put me on 6-Mercaptopurine, also known as 6-MP.

I read enough about 6-MP to realize that it was a drug used for acute lymphoblastic leukemia, and that told me all I needed to know. It was a pretty serious drug. *I guess my condition is pretty serious,* I thought. I only received a fraction of what chemo patients receive and was experiencing severe nausea, bruising, exhaustion, fatigue, and the incredible ability to fall into a deep sleep like a hibernating bear. That was the scariest part to me—not being able to wake up. I remember one morning my dog came up and put his snout between my nose and my mouth, checking to make sure I was still alive as I hadn't moved for hours. I wasn't sure if I would wake up if the house was on fire, but that was nothing in comparison to the possible liver toxicity that met me a few months later.

When I was first put on 6-MP, my gastroenterologist told me that I would need to get my bloodwork done once a month. Being the ignorant twenty-five-year-old that I was, I had no idea why I needed to get my bloodwork done once a month. This quickly changed when my liver enzymes were off the charts a few months later, indicating possible hepatotoxicity.

Oh great, I thought. *Not only has this drug made me super nauseous, has hardly contained my colitis symptoms, but now might have screwed up my liver? That's just freaking fantastic. AAAHHHH!!!!* My gastroenterologist immediately took me off 6-MP and told me I needed to get my blood drawn once a week until my liver enzymes returned to normal. It took six months for my liver enzymes to return to normal, and thank goodness they did, because if they hadn't, I would've needed a liver biopsy.

I was so blown away. First, I was shitting blood out of my ass, then was put on the 'roids to try and fix that, which, in turn, transformed me into a fat psycho-bitch. When my gastroenterologist decided to stop the 'roid treatment, he put me on 6-MP. While on the 6-MP, I was still experiencing symptoms, though not as severe, but couldn't really do anything because I was too exhausted, too nauseous, and all the while, my liver was, unbeknownst to me, slowly getting screwed up?! What the hell was going on? Aren't these drugs supposed to help, not hurt? *This is some screwed up shit*, I thought to myself, no pun intended.

After my 6-MP scare and two years after my initial diagnosis, my gastroenterologist decided that the next step for me was Remicade, a drug in the biologic category. This would be my first intravenous drug therapy and I would have to go to an infusion center to receive my treatment. I used to refer to Remicade as my "mouse juice" as it has mouse-human antibodies. After the initial dosage, I received an infusion once every eight weeks.

The first time I arrived at the ambulatory infusion center, I was given a humbling and sobering reality check almost instantly. While receiving my infusion, I often sat next to patients receiving chemotherapy. I learned the importance of life sitting next to people literally fighting for their lives. I, yet again, learned that life is fragile, and that the human spirit is unbreakable.

I once sat in an infusion room with three remarkable individuals I will never forget. The first was a man sitting to my right, Mr. Akre, who was fifty-nine years young. I quickly learned that he was suffering from lung cancer, had graduated from the same university I did, spent his career as a military officer, and had a thirty-one-year-old daughter who had just started her own business. He told me that he was excited for her and hoped to see her prosper. We talked about his cancer when he told me, "They gave me seven to twelve." I stopped talking for a moment, completely dumbfounded.

Not sure what I just heard, I carefully replied, "Wait, you've got seven to twelve months left on chemo?"

"To live," he replied.

At that moment, my heart bled for this man. I could not even imagine what he was going through. "Don't listen to them," I began. "They don't know. YOU will be the anomaly." Mr. Akre smiled.

We started discussing the side effects of chemo and he said, "Even if the chemo makes me really ill, I'll do it because if it gives me one more month, it's worth it."

Then the man sitting to my left piped in, "Ten years ago, they gave me six months to live. I'm still alive today." He then went on to explain that he was diagnosed with a rare form of cancer called liposarcoma ten years prior. At the time of his diagnosis, there were only seventy-four documented cases of that particular cancer in the world. He was given an "expiration date," as he put it, by his doctors. Yet, he defied all odds, showing the strength of the human spirit.

His comment led to a room-wide discussion (three chemo patients, two men, one woman, and our nurse were in the room with me). We all agreed that life-changing day that we were all fighters and would not be beaten by our illnesses. We laughed and joked. Mr. Akre joked that he had paid into social security his entire adult life and would be damned if he didn't see any of that money! The man to my left joked that when he first married his wife after he was diagnosed with cancer, he told her that she didn't have to worry about him dying because he didn't want her to be happy a day of her life, and by him dying, she would be happy. Our room erupted with laughter. Through all of the pain, suffering and cheating death, we laughed. Our room was so loud that we could be heard down the hallway. There was faith and hope in our infusion room that day. The woman in the room, though I never learned what her illness was, laughed and felt the positive spirit that arose us all.

From that point forward, every infusion I went to, I would meditate and think positive thoughts, desperately hoping that this drug would heal the ulcers in my colon. On November 26th, 2008, it finally did. I was on Remicade for seven months before I officially went into remission, which was nearly two years and six months after my initial diagnosis. My gastroenterologist also had to give me the maximum dosage my body could handle. Lucky for me, I was able to enjoy remission for a year. It was so weird to experience, and I was so thankful.

Even while I was in remission, I came to resent Remicade. I got sick and tired of having a suppressed immune system. I no longer wanted the toxic load of Mickey Mouse coursing through my veins. I wanted to give my body a chance to go medicine-free, just to see what it would do.

I believe the majority of patients who give a damn struggle with having to take immunosuppressant medications. It freakin' sucks, but is sometimes necessary. I struggle to this day with the fact that I have been on immunosuppressant therapy since 2006. When I was close to being completely off my meds, I was thrown a curve ball during my third pregnancy and had to begin taking Humira. While pregnant. Definitely not the medicine-free life, or pregnancy, I had imagined. Prior to my third pregnancy, I was on an extremely low dose of azathioprine (50mg) and

Lialda and felt like it was only a matter of months until I would be able to finally go medication-free. Trust me, I would love to be completely off the medicine, and I truly believe I will get there when my body is ready.

The best advice I can give is to be your very own *patient matter expert*. If your doctor recommends a drug that you aren't comfortable with, ask questions, read medical and scientific journals, research all the options, talk to others that have been on those medications, and express your concerns to your healthcare team. Trust me, I 100% understand that being told by your doc that you may need to take an injection, such as Cimzia or Humira, or an infusion, such as Remicade, is freaking scary. But so is crapping lots of blood, not being able to control your bowels, and possibly dying of malnourishment (which almost happened to me).

Do your homework and educate yourself as much as you can. When I was first put on Remicade, I was too naïve to ask questions. In the end, I would have ended up on Remicade anyway because long term use of prednisone just wasn't feasible for me. It was then that I realized that sometimes you have to take a potent drug to get your body where it needs to be. Just because you are on a biologic or immunosuppressant now doesn't mean, in my opinion, that you will be on it for the rest of your life. It is simply a means to an end. So, seriously, keep the faith, and do your homework on the different drug options available to you!

Doggy Style

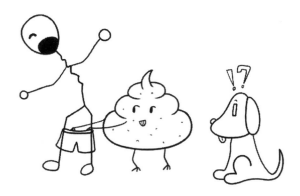

One warm June night, my considerate 110 pound German Shepherd woke me up at 3:30am because he wasn't feeling well and his little sphincter was telling him he needed to have a wonderful stroll of 'rhea in the woods or it was going to end up all over my carpet. I reluctantly got out of bed, put his collar on him, walked out the door, and off he ran into the woods behind my neighbor's house.

I patiently waited for him when BAM!!! I got hit with intense cramping and knew that I needed to run across the street and park my bum on the closest toilet in my house, but I couldn't because my dog was having his 'rhea in the woods and was nowhere to be seen! If I ran across the street and left him alone, it was certain he would run away for a midnight stroll.

At that moment, *my* sphincter began to quiver. I broke out into a cold sweat, clenched my butt cheeks together as tight as I could, and hoped with all my might that I could keep this poo inside my colon. Up to this point, I had never experienced the pleasure of crapping myself. I knew that the urgent cramping meant an urgent need to find a bathroom, but I also knew I didn't want to deal with a lost dog!!

The cramping got so intense that I finally couldn't hold it anymore. A gush of warm liquid filled my panties, and I prayed it wouldn't run down my leg and soak through my bright purple and pink fleece pajama bottoms. OH. MY. GOSH. I *just* crapped myself! Here I was, in the middle of the night, standing in front of my neighbor's house, covered in my own shit, not knowing what the hell to do next. I couldn't wrap my head around the fact that I had literally just crapped myself!

About thirty seconds later, my dog ran back to me. He stopped, and with a confused face, started sniffing in the air, trying to find the source of the stink. He then looked at me, slowly walked over, and carefully sniffed me from my nether regions all the way down to my ankles. A look of confusion flooded his furry little face. *Yes, you asshole dog! I shit my pants so you wouldn't shit your fur! Except you're smarter than me in this instant because you shit in the bushes! Show a little sympathy and gratitude here and stop embarrassing me even more!!*

But then it hit me! DAMN! Why hadn't I been smart enough to go doggy style?! My dog was smart enough to shit in the woods. Why didn't that idea occur to me too?! Yeah, it would have been awkward if my neighbor woke up and caught me popping a squat in the trees, but hey, it would be even more awkward if my neighbor woke up and came out of his house to talk to me only to discover that I was standing there in panties full of shit!

If that ever happened to me now, I'd pick the biggest freaking tree and shit behind it! Also, if I knew I was flaring, I'd carry around some toilet paper just in case. With this disease, you have got to throw conventional thinking out the window and get creative! Should this ever happen to you, I recommend going doggy style! It's much easier than throwing a pair of panties away, rinsing off your favorite jammie bottoms, and having to explain to your dog why you aren't creative enough to shit like they do.

Truly shitting your pants for the first time is extremely hard to grasp. It goes against absolutely everything that became second nature to you once you stopped pissing in diapers as a baby. In our society, and pretty much in all societies, it is *not normal* and *extremely embarrassing* to shit your pants!

After this incident happened, I slowly walked back to my house and immediately burst into tears once I got inside. I could not believe what had just happened! I, as a 24-year-old beautiful, strong woman, had just shit my pants. In front of my neighbor's yard. It was more than I could bear. I carefully took off my jammies and panties, rolled them up, and triple bagged them in plastic bags. *Sayonara, favorite jammies. Sorry you met your demise in the messy way that you did,* I thought to myself.

To top it all off, this happened three months after I was newly diagnosed with ulcerative colitis and my husband was three months into a six month military deployment. I was alone, sick, in denial about my diagnosis, and at times, extremely depressed. For the first time in my life, I felt true hopelessness.

A few weeks later, on a warm August afternoon, I was laying on my bed with the worst headache I've ever experienced thanks to the cocktail of medicines that I was on. I remember staring at my big black and tan German Shepherd, Caesar, sleeping peacefully and thinking, *My dog is going to outlive me. I doubt I'll even make it to thirty.* I actually *believed* those thoughts because I was *that sick,* but I never let that show on the outside to others.

Every day, I would go to work with a smile on my face and, with the exception of constantly rushing to the bathroom, I continued on as if nothing traumatic was happening in my gut. I went out with friends, partied, ate whatever I wanted as I had not quite figured out the food-body connection, and tried to be as "normal" as possible. I tried to be the same "me" that I was before my diagnosis. On the surface, I appeared normal, as if this disease was just a tiny bump in the road and not a major life-changing event. That's how I tried to play it off anyway.

I would joke with my friends and coworkers about shitting blood, stating it really wasn't that bad, just a little inconvenient. I successfully played it off like I was perfectly fine and that nothing was really happening to me, but those were all lies.

Something major was wreaking havoc on my gut, and I was in absolute denial. Instead of admitting that I was extremely ill, I would go on compulsive shopping trips, eat as much junk as I wanted, drink a little too much, and party even harder. I would do everything and anything to keep from admitting that I felt as though I was dying on the inside due to the agonizing physical and mental pain caused by my ulcerated colon.

This self-denial landed me in the hospital five months after my initial diagnosis. My husband was still gone, I downplayed the hospitalization to my family, and the only visitors I had were a few coworkers, a priest, and maybe one or two acquaintances. Even then, I did not *accept* the magnitude of the situation before me. I was unwilling to admit that I was extremely ill, that I felt the loneliest I had ever felt in my life, and that neither my family nor friends understood what was happening to my body.

Everybody has a breaking point, and I was about to break. A few weeks after being released from the hospital, I could no longer take the severity of my illness, could no longer take the drugs coursing through my veins, and could no longer take the extreme isolation that I felt. It is really hard to appear normal on the outside when your insides are, quite literally, tearing themselves apart.

My colon was ulcerated, my body was "puffy" due to the prednisone, my life was a mess, I didn't feel as though I had a support system, and I could no longer take the unknown demons that were wreaking havoc on my life—a life that was once so full of promise. I fell to my knees, sobbing uncontrollably, and for the first time in my life, contemplated suicide. I *could not* take it anymore.

In the deepest, darkest moment of my life, God sent me a sign. My dog, Caesar, ran up to me and started licking the tears from my face. I desperately hugged him and sobbed uncontrollably. I couldn't believe that I was actually contemplating suicide. That was so *not me.* I cried until I could no longer cry as exhaustion once again took over my body. When I loosened my grip on Caesar, his neck was soaked and I had black fur matted on the side of my face. But Caesar saved me that night. Thanks to Caesar, who I believe is an angel from above, I knew that somehow, someway, I would get through this. I had no idea how or when I would get through this difficult time in my life as I no longer knew who I was and simply couldn't wrap my head around what was happening to me, but I had faith that it would somehow happen.

My husband came home a month later and was shocked by my drastic physical and personality change. He had briefly seen me two months prior when his submarine pulled into a domestic port and I was at an unhealthy 105 pounds. Now, here I was, standing before him, at 130 pounds, puffed up from prednisone. As far as personality goes, he was used to me being optimistic, funny, and generally always in a good mood. When he came home, I was extremely moody, exhausted, and beaten to the core of my soul. *I was beaten to the core of my soul.* The house reflected how I felt as it was messy and unkempt. My diet was a disaster. My life was a disaster. I was a disaster.

Ignoring the disease once again caught up to me. Instead of facing and accepting the disease, I pushed away those who cared about me most. My husband, parents, and friends were pushed away. They didn't understand what I was going through, so why should I deal with them? I was *done explaining myself.* I got tired of questions and comments from family like, "Why are you flaring?" or, "You shouldn't eat that," or, "What did you do to flare? You *must have done something* to get sick again," or, "What did you eat? That's probably why you're sick." And comments from friends like, "Why can't you just stay healthy?" or, "Why can't you go out with us?" or, "You're so boring now."

In short, I could no longer take the "it's your fault" stigma that I felt was being put on me *every time* I started flaring, which, for the first year after being diagnosed, was every other month. I was tired of fighting with my husband. All he wanted was for me to live a healthier lifestyle to help minimize or possibly prevent symptoms, but I was resistant and pushed him away.

I felt the weight of the world on my shoulders, so I told him I wanted a divorce. That, ladies and gents, is when the ball dropped.

He begged me to go to counseling, and I reluctantly agreed. In my mind, my true decision to leave him was already made, but I thought I'd go through the motions so I wouldn't appear heartless. I figured that I might as well exhaust all resources so I would never look back and regret any decisions made. It took one and *only one* session for me to realize that I was about to make the worst decision of my life. I realized that my husband had been the only true cheerleader by my side, and that the reason I was pushing him away was because I didn't feel like I deserved him. I realized that I was so angry that the disease had taken over my life that I didn't feel like I deserved love or happiness.

I hated myself for being sick, though getting sick was completely out of my control and not my choosing by a longshot. I realized that the true reason I wanted to leave was because I didn't want to burden him with a sick version of myself. He married one person, and the disease had turned me into another. I felt as though he married a lemon, not the strong, healthy, athletic, vibrant woman he initially planned to live his life with. It was then that I realized that I needed to dig the *shit* out of my mind, body, and soul so that my true healing journey could begin.

I needed to release the baggage so that my colon could begin to heal. I never realized that past pain I had suppressed for years was contributing to my disease. I needed to work at releasing the hurt and pain that I had been carrying around on my shoulders for years. My pain went much deeper than I imagined, and thanks to my husband, who refused to give up on me, I realized that. I saw, right before me, unconditional love. It was that day, the day of our first and last counseling session, that I realized I was worthy, even though I was sick. It was then that I also put my stilettos and martini glasses aside and decided to fully commit to my healing journey.

All the Rage (Not in a Good Way)

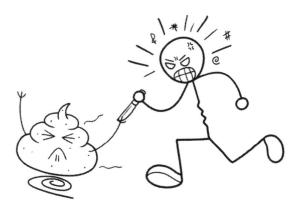

I had never heard of prednisone prior to being diagnosed with ulcerative colitis. I had heard of 'roid rage, but that was more to do with the anabolic steroids that crazy body builders use to get buff super quickly. I had heard of the 'roid rage that they experienced, but always thought that was bullshit.

It took me a hot minute to figure out that prednisone is in the corticosteroid family, which is completely different than anabolic 'roids. They are completely different! Plus, my use was completely involuntary!! I *had* to take prednisone to keep me from having explosive bloody 'rhea!

What I didn't bank on was the extreme weight gain, night sweats, not being able to sleep, serious mood swings, irritability toward those around me, and just plain old-fashioned rage. That's right. Rage! I "heard" that 'roid rage was real, but like I said, I thought it was bullshit!! Boy, oh boy, was I wrong!

I was immediately put on prednisone in 2006 after my ulcerative colitis diagnosis. I didn't think much of it, or the side effects, until the night I turned into a crazy, insane, Tasmanian devil meets the Incredible Hulk sociopath.

It was the first night my husband left on deployment, so I was sleeping alone in our bedroom with my brother sleeping in the guest bedroom down the hall. Our bedroom window overlooked the front of the house, including the driveway. At approximately 3am, I awoke to what sounded like commotion outside. *There is NO WAY anybody is out there. You're just hearing things,* I thought to myself. I looked out the window anyway and saw two low-lifes on both sides of my husband's car, trying to break in. For the first time in my life, I saw red. The color red literally flashed before my eyes and I was instantly filled with rage. *OH, HELL NO!* I thought as I sprinted out of the bedroom with only a sports bra and underwear on. On my way out, I flipped the staircase light on so I wouldn't trip down the stairs, opened the front door, and ran outside. The two would-be car thieves were running down the street, so what did I do? The totally rational thing of course. *I chased them.* I had no weapon to protect myself, hardly any clothes on, but the rage of a gazillion tiny Spartans burning within me. I finally gave up on my chase and walked home. When I got there, my brother was staring at me in complete confusion and horror. Was it because I was in my undies and sports bra? Probably. I would be scarred for life if I saw him running down the street in his tighty-whities. It wasn't until then that I realized I had acted both irrationally and dangerously. I could have been seriously hurt, but I didn't think about that because all I saw and *felt* was red. It took a few days for me to realize how stupidly I had acted. I laughed it off when I told people the story, but truth be told, it scared me to think that I acted so impulsively and with such anger.

After the car incident, I did not experience true 'roid rage until six months later when my husband returned home from his six month deployment. I was used to making all the decisions solo and had my routine down to a T. What happens when you throw another person in the mix with a ticking time bomb? An explosion, of course!

My husband was only home for two weeks when I completely lost it on him. We had a minor disagreement, but in my mind, it was a really huge disagreement (though it was probably over something as silly as should we go out to eat pumpkin pancakes or should we make them from home?). We were standing face to face. I instantly went from 0% angry to 100% psycho, pushed him down onto the couch, stomped up the stairs, threw the laundry basket down the stairs, punched the wall while letting out a roar of true anger, stomped into the master bathroom, shut and locked the door, and began sobbing uncontrollably. I was *so mad* at him, but it didn't make any sense. I couldn't believe my actions. They were so violent and *so out of character* for me! What happened to the easy going, fun-loving girl I used to be? It was scary to think that I could turn into a complete monster with the flip of a switch!! My confused thoughts were interrupted when I heard my husband lightly knock on the door, saying, "Emma, will you please come out of there?!"

"NO!" I screamed, probably more out of embarrassment than rage.

Eventually, I made it out of the bathroom, fell into his arms crying a sea of tears, telling him I didn't know what was wrong with me. I told him I felt like a complete monster and had trouble controlling anger that I never knew I could possess.

"You're not a monster," he gently responded. I held onto him for what felt like an eternity, trying to figure out where to go from there.

I'm embarrassed to admit that nobody was immune from my rage, though my family got the brunt of it. Caesar, my precious dog, wasn't spared either. There were times I would get so angry at him for no apparent reason that he would run away from me and hide. Talk about hitting a new level of crazy when I realized my 110 pound German Shepherd was hiding from me because he wasn't sure what the hell I was going to do!!!

My parents, well, they experienced my rage too. I distinctly remember driving to get ice-cream on a warm Arizona summer evening. My dad, mom, niece and I were in a very good mood, chatting away, without a care in the world. I was in the driver's seat, and when we were close to home, my dad tried to give me instructions on how to pull into the driveway as it was a bit tricky. I had to go up a tiny curb and revved the car, but it wouldn't climb over the curb. "Give it more gas," he instructed.

"No!" I exploded back. "It doesn't want to climb the stupid curb. If you want it done, *you* do it yourself. This is ridiculous." With that, I stormed out of the car, running and all, leaving my parents and niece staring at each other, in complete shock by my actions. I apologized a few hours later and they understood that those actions were not my norm, but it still weighed on my mind. *I have got to get a grip before people no longer want to be around me,* I thought to myself.

As I tapered off of the prednisone, the "psycho-bitch" in me slowly disappeared. I returned back to my normal "nicest person in the world" self that people described me as. It was amazing how much better my psyche felt when I was off the 'roids. I felt like *me* again; no longer a super pissed off version of the girl I "once knew."

It took *several* on-off prednisone treatments for me to realize how to handle my irrational anger. Or, more importantly, how not to act on it. Finally, after being on-and-off the prednisone gravy train for three years, I told my husband that I would no longer act out in anger when I was on the 'roids because it wasn't fair to him or me. Instead, I would just stop talking if I got really mad about something.

The no-talking-when-irrationally-mad approach worked, but was super hard for me to follow through with and keep under control. I had a constant struggle with a demon on one shoulder and an angel on the other. The somewhat tempting demon encouraged me to just scream out and tell my husband how pissed I was, how mad I was at him, and that every little thing that pissed me off (for no reason) was all his fault! It constantly felt like this little demon was yelling, "Let out the bottled rage that is coursing through your veins!! You'll feel so much better to just let it out! Who cares how he feels?!" The angel, on the other hand, kept repeating to me, "You are being completely irrational. You know you are being irrational. Keep calm, keep it together. You know your anger right now is completely irrational." This back-and-forth usually resulted in tears, but at least I didn't explode on those that matter the most to me.

I'm here to tell you, to this day, I still have a love-hate relationship with prednisone. I've had more than my fair share of oral and intravenous steroids. I am also forever indebted to the intravenous steroids for saving not only my colon, but my life. It doesn't get any more serious than that.

The struggle is real! Though prednisone has given me my quality of life back when flaring, it has also presented new challenges. Gaining weight while on the 'roids is hard to deal with, especially when it's twenty-five pounds over the course of two months. More notably, it was really hard to be on prednisone for FIVE MONTHS after giving birth to my daughter. I was still, almost two years later, trying to lose that mess!

Though feeling like the marshmallow man from *Ghost Busters* is real, it is nothing compared to the rage that you may experience. Please, for the sake of those around you, recognize it for what it is—irrational thinking and anger—and don't act on it! Find your outlet, whether it be running, cycling, painting, journaling, and release your anger there. Those around you will thank you, and you won't feel like a dumbass, apologizing for not being able to control your emotions. Steroids suck, but are sometimes a necessary evil.

Shit Show

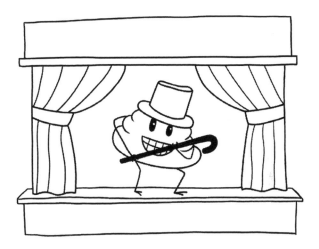

About two years after getting diagnosed, I packed up my dog and drove to Arizona to spend six months with my parents. My husband had just left on his second deployment since my diagnosis and would be unreachable and out of the country for the next seven months. I was on Remicade, still flaring, and not in the best mental health. I had just lost my job due to my diagnosis changing from ulcerative colitis to Crohn's disease and was in no condition to commit to another job anytime soon.

Shortly after arriving at my parents' house, my brother let me know that he would have his boss over for an early morning meeting the following day. The meeting was to take place down the hall from the room I was staying in. No big deal, right? Ha! I wasn't so lucky. Unbeknownst to me, my colon had a party planned, and I was going to be the life of the party...

The next morning, I awoke, heard the meeting between my brother and his boss going on down the hall, and instantaneously got hit with super intense cramping. This was the kind of cramping that meant *you better get your arse to the bathroom or you're going to shit all over yourself!* I jumped out of bed, sprinted down the hall, all while trying to squeeze my sphincter to keep me from embarrassing myself in front of my brother and his boss. Running down the hall, I remember thinking, *Please-oh-please-oh-please just let me get there! Oh gosh, it hurts. Oh no, oh no, it's coming out. SHIT!!!!!!!!*

I slammed the bathroom door, sat on the toilet as fast as I could, and let the humiliation flow. Not only did I *not* make it to the bathroom, but I also managed to get bloody shit all over the floor and create a smell that would be fitting for an emergency room scenario. I was SO embarrassed. SO humiliated. I broke into tears, feeling less than human. What the hell was happening to me? I couldn't even have the dignity of controlling my sphincter. I thought, *Thanks, asshole. Oh wait, no thanks. You're fucking useless.*

Through a sea of tears, I remember my teenage niece opening the door. I embarrassingly looked up and asked her to shut the door in a quiet and defeated tone. She was so compassionate and just wanted to know if I needed any help cleaning up the mess. I sobbed even harder. I was *so embarrassed.* I felt *so powerless. So humiliated.* So *out of control.* I thanked her for her offering to help, but declined the offer. This shit show was mine, and mine only to clean.

I cleaned myself up, bleached the shit out of the floor (literally), and showered again. Once I pulled myself together enough to come out of the bathroom, I remember my brother walking down the hall asking, "What the fuck happened earlier and what smells so bad down here?!" I lost it again. It turns out that he and his boss heard *everything*. I hid in the bathroom, sobbing uncontrollably. I couldn't control ANYTHING. My emotions were a mess, my bowels were a mess, and my life was in total disarray. I didn't understand what I'd done to deserve such humiliation. I felt completely defeated, disgusting, and hopeless. At the ripe ol' age of twenty-six, I didn't have a lot of hope for the future.

Once I gathered my emotions, I took a deep breath and left the bathroom that had stripped me of so much dignity that morning. I called my doctor, told him I needed some prednisone, that the Remicade still wasn't working, and that shit had just hit the floor. I was hanging on by a thread. I was scared and had no idea what the future held for me.

Looking back, I wish I could have been strong enough to check my defeated emotions, humiliation, and feelings of hopelessness on the bathroom floor as I walked out that depressing morning. But I wasn't ready to give up control and accept what was happening to my body. I was angry, depressed, and still wondering *why* this disease had chosen me, and *why* I had to put up with it when all my peers were moving on with their careers and lives. I didn't like that I had to worry about shitting my pants every time I left the house. I wondered what it would be like to walk out of the house while flaring and not have to worry about losing control of my bowels. I didn't accept the disease for what it was, and that was the problem. I was letting the bloody shit show that unfolded on the bathroom floor that morning define me. I wish, at that time, I would have accepted that the unpredictability and lack of control that comes with this disease does not define me. Just like it does not define you. It is not who you are deep in your soul.

Unfortunately, my friends, at some point, you will more than likely lose control of your bowels. But that is okay. *It is not* who you are, it is just something that you have to deal with. It will get better. I promise. Remember, perfectly healthy people shit their pants too. As embarrassing, soul-sucking moments come, let them happen, learn from them, check them at the door (or floor), and let them go.

Now, several years later, I could care less that I lost total control that morning. I draw strength from that moment, have learned from it, and am a better person for it. This may seem so cliché, but one day, you will look back at your most embarrassing moments and laugh.

Luau Poo - Wow

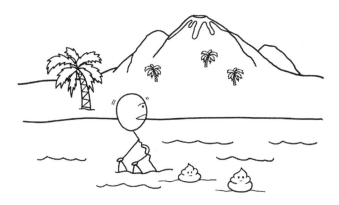

In June of 2010, I went on a family vacation to Kauai. I'd been looking forward to this trip all year, worked hard to get the highly sought after bikini body, and was ready to show off my assets…except for the fact that, in May, my asshole started exploding and didn't want to be shown off. Wow, totally inconvenient. I had two choices. I could stay at home and lick my wounds *or* I could get creative!

On the way to the airport, which was about an hour drive, we had to stop three times at less than ideal gas stations so I could crap. I'm living proof that in the world of Crohn's and colitis, there is no such thing as a gas station bathroom phobia! This wasn't the way I envisioned my vacation starting, but I rolled with it. Thanks to not eating or drinking anything on the plane, my flight was uneventful. We landed in Kauai and I was ready for vacation to begin! I would do whatever I needed to do to make this trip work.

My family went to the beach A LOT. I remember passing the bathroom as we walked through the entryway of each beach we visited and refused to camp out not only in front of the bathroom, but at the entryway of the beach. I needed quiet and solace. I wanted to get as far away from people as possible so I could finally relax, calm my nerves and anxiety, and shit in peace if need be. If my lower abdominals felt the intense cramping of inevitable shit, my plan was to run like Jackie Joyner-Kersee to the ocean, swim like Michael Phelps, and dump my shit in the ocean, three nautical miles be damned! Sorry, Clean Water Act. My point is, I was willing to do whatever I needed to do to enjoy some sort of normalcy, and sunbathing and enjoying the ocean were my highest priority! Thankfully, I never had to test out my ocean shit escape plan. I'm pretty sure the fish are still thanking me to this day.

I digress. The part of vacation I remember most is when my parents thought it was a fantastic idea to get tickets for a luau on the complete *opposite* end of the island. And to top it off, they thought it would be genius to rent a party bus that would also be full of other partying luau-goers to take us there so we could all drink and not have to worry about driving back. Um, wrong answer Mom and Dad! I pretty much gave up drinking once I committed to my healing journey because I realized that alcohol made my flares much worse and was pretty much one of the worst things I could put into my body. I also didn't want to have to shit in the tiny bathroom of a tour bus full of partying luau-goers. I did, however, take comfort in the fact that there would be a bathroom on the party bus, as tiny as it might be. Or so I thought.

When the big purple party bus arrived, I slowly walked up the steps, looked right at the bus driver and said, "You have bathrooms back there, right?"

His reply, "Yeah, but they are out of service."

Starting to sweat and panic, I replied, "What do you mean out of service? Like, they're broken?"

His reply, "They aren't working."

I nervously went to my seat and sat down. This "party" bus ride just went from miserable to downright scary. What would I do if I had to shit? Yell at him to pull the bus over? Hell no! My plan B was simple. I'd run my ass down the aisle, open the door to the "out of service" bathroom, and shit if I have to! That was a much better option than possibly crapping myself in my seat or attempting to make it to a gas station bathroom after a huge bus took forever to pull over and park. I would lose in either of those scenarios.

Thankfully, I arrived at the luau with no poo incidents and was actually able to enjoy the luau with no cramping or crapping! Hallelujah! Except, in the back of my mind, I was nervous about the bus ride home. When the time came, I reluctantly loaded the party bus to start the torturous trek across the island to our condo. I hoped to God that the small quantity of food I ate at the luau would not cause me to cramp or my sphincter to freak, with the result of me having to crap in the "out of service" bathroom. I'm a little bit of a rebel, but didn't want to deal with the hassle of explaining to the driver why I used his "out of service, but not really" toilet. However, it would have served him right…jerk!

I stared out the window on the ride home as people around me excitedly chatted about the luau. I wondered what it would be like to not have to worry about always being paranoid about being around a bathroom. As I watched the lights pass by, I looked into the dark sky and, for a split second, wondered what it would be like to be normal. Realizing that those thoughts were neither healthy nor conducive to healing, I let them go. I needed to remember and embrace that I was my own normal. Even if *my normal* meant shitting in an off-limits toilet. Thankfully, that night did not turn into a luau poo-wow as I never once had any poo incidents. I think having a "poo emergency plan" for each potentially embarrassing situation stopped the flare fairy from messing with my mind, hence preventing an embarrassing moment.

When flaring, having a plan that calms the nerves is one of the best things you can do for yourself. We definitely can't control every situation we will be in, but we can improvise when in less than ideal situations. It is important to go about your life, whether that be going to your child's soccer game, shopping with friends, or going on an amazing date with the guy/gal of your dreams. Just have your emergency plan if need be. To this day, I am glad I went on our annual family vacation. It was extremely stressful at times, and wondering if I was going to have to shit in less than ideal circumstances was always in the back of my mind. But I was out and about anyway because that was better than being chained to the toilet.

After my diagnosis, I acknowledged that my parents were scared and struggling with the fact that their daughter was diagnosed with a chronic illness that they could do absolutely nothing about. I also acknowledged that they desperately wanted to erase any and all remnants of the ulcerations that had not only taken over my colon, but had taken over my life. I know that if they had it their way, they would take the disease on themselves so I would no longer suffer. But that's not how life works, and certainly isn't how Crohn's disease or ulcerative colitis works.

Instead of taking personally the somewhat ignorant but well-meaning comments family and friends said, I started a blog about my daily life with ulcerative colitis to educate them so they could better understand the disease along with my daily struggles and tiny victories. I wanted them to realize that this beast of a diagnosis was my cross to bear and my journey to undertake, and that they were going to have to check their criticisms and opinions at the door.

I tried to keep my blog current so I didn't have to continuously repeat myself each time I spoke on the phone with a friend or family member. The infamous question of, "How are you feeling?" every time I spoke with a well-meaning friend or family member over the phone started to wear on me. The last thing I wanted to do was talk about not being able to control my bowels and shitting blood in the toilet. I, instead, informed them about my blog and told them anything and everything about my current state of illness could be found there. I just wanted to talk about non-disease related topics, but I knew they were worried and only had the best intentions at heart. Had situations been reversed, I would have done the same, so again, I can't fault them.

To the friends and family of those suffering from inflammatory bowel disease, or any chronic illness for that matter, I encourage you to not make their illness the focal point of any conversation. Those suffering from a chronic disease live it day-in and day-out, and would love any normalcy to any conversation. As a good rule of thumb, think of what your conversations were like pre-diagnosis and use that as a reference point! Instead of their individual illness being the focal point of every conversation, I encourage you to discuss things that have absolutely nothing to do with their disease or current state of health. It's totally fine to express your concern and support, but try to not focus on their illness! It will go a long way overall!

To those living with a chronic illness day-in and day-out, hang in there! If you feel certain family members or friends are not being supportive or are constantly criticizing you, it is 100% okay to drop them like a two-ton rock! Sometimes you outgrow your friends, especially those that are non-supportive or won't take the time to listen or empathize with your disease. It doesn't matter if you've been friends since childhood; you have to let go of those that bring you down! What is most important is to minimize stress and surround yourself with a tribe of individuals full of nothing but love and support for you! A strong tribe will help you in your darkest and toughest moments.

Stage Fright

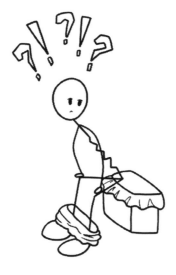

My husband and I were living in Washington State when his five-year high school reunion invitation was sent out via Facebook. Unfortunately for me, my husband went to high school in Washington State, which meant we were going to make an appearance. What's the last thing anybody wants to do when flaring? Oh, yeah, go to a high school reunion with a bunch of people you don't even know! However, being the supportive wife I am, I told my husband we could absolutely go and that I would be fine, though I was having ten to fifteen explosive bloody bowel movements a day. I have no idea if I was in a state of stubbornness or denial, but regardless, I was not going to let the disease hold me back from a night of non-drunken stupor with folks I neither knew nor would probably ever see again.

The evening of the reunion, I pulled on my favorite designer jeans, buttoned my silk tank top, put on my three-inch wedges, and was ready to rock. My grandma, who was visiting at the time, snapped a picture of my hubby and I as we were on our way out the door. *Damn, we look good,* I thought as we walked out the door.

The reunion was thirty minutes away, and the trip was uneventful until we were *two minutes* away from the venue and on an extremely busy road that paralleled a neighborhood full of houses. I remember thinking that it was a nice neighborhood when, out of nowhere, my lower abdominals started intensely cramping and I felt as though I was getting stabbed in the gut by some invisible entity. I looked at my husband in horror and yelled, "Pull the car over. I have to shit!"

"Now? We're only two minutes away!"

"NOW! I'm not going to make it!" I screamed in terror.

He pulled the car over and I instantly jumped out to grab my makeshift paper bag toilet from the trunk. After I grabbed my "toilet," I ran to the passenger-side door, all while staring at the houses, praying to God that nobody could see my tiny white ass from their windows. *This can't be happening,* I thought. *This is so humiliating. I really, really hope nobody sees me through their windows.*

Using the passenger-side door as my "privacy" door, I pulled my designer jeans down, squatted in my wedges, and was ready for the humiliation to begin. A flood of thoughts took over my already fragile mind and I began thinking, *Please, don't splatter all over yourself. I can't believe I'm actually using my makeshift toilet. Thank God I had it in the trunk. High five to me. This really sucks big, fat, hairy balls. Shit, I hope nobody is looking out their window. This is so freaking embarrassing. Damn me for being too arrogant. I am so humiliated.*

Then it hit me. For the *first* time in my life, my colon and sphincter got stage fright. This was the first and *only time* I have never had an uncontrollable bowel movement after experiencing intense cramping and sphincter spasms. I was blown away.

"Emma, are you okay?" my husband asked. I pulled up my jeans, fixed my shirt, and looked at him in complete awe.

"My ass got stage fright," I told him in disbelief. He sympathetically stared at me, not sure what to say next.

I threw my toilet in the backseat, sat down in the passenger seat, and while counting my blessings, began to giggle. In an unsure tone, I said, "A freaking miracle. My asshole got stage fright! I have *no idea* what just happened."

As we drove off, I stared at the houses, wondering if anybody had seen my tiny white ass. We made it to the reunion, and for the rest of the evening, my colon was completely dormant—no lower abdominal cramping, no urgency issues, nothing, nada, zip. I spent the rest of the evening in shock, not quite knowing what to make of the stage fright me and my colon experienced.

To this day, I still have no idea what happened. I am thankful for not shitting in my makeshift toilet right next to several houses, possibly scarring families and small dogs for life. I am thankful I was prepared with my toilet. And I laugh at my own arrogance as I walked out of the house that evening knowing for sure that I wouldn't possibly crap my pants because I "looked too good." Bullshit. The disease doesn't discriminate, but it sure as hell didn't rear its ugly head that evening.

Perhaps it was because I was prepared with a toilet in my car, so that eased *some* anxiety. I'll never know. The only recommendation I can give to others is to always be prepared for the inevitable, carry your toilet of choice in your trunk, and get out and party hardy, even if it's with a bunch of strangers you don't know or won't ever see again.

▬ ▬ ▬ / ▪ ▬ ▮▮▮ ▰▰ ▬ / ▪ ▬ ▬ ▮▮▮ ▮▮▮ ▰▰ ▬

2010 is a year that will go down in the history books for me. According to the zodiac calendar, it was the year of the tiger. This seemed quite appropriate as the flare born in my gut that year was definitely reminiscent of a tiger. It almost killed me by slowly sneaking up on me and then tearing me apart piece by piece, bit by bit.

For me, the year of the tiger kicked off in late January with a minor flare. My symptoms were very mild bloody poo, sometimes only mucous, but nothing uncontrollable. My sphincter was playing nice, so I was able to keep the flare in check with diet, yoga, meditation, Remicade, and plenty of rest. This flare was manageable until May, when I got food poisoning from an undercooked piece of chicken. Little did I know that damn piece of pollo was going to make me loco over the next nine months! Read on for all the dirty details, my friends! The worst is yet to come.

The Curious Case of the Shitties

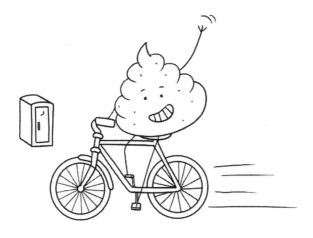

When my body starts flaring, the flare usually starts mildly with some blood in my poo and slowly works its way up to being a bit more urgent, eventually leading to not only severe cramping but several bouts of uncontrollable bloody 'rhea on a daily basis. But before this freakin' crime scene happens, my colon usually gives me a heads up. I know what to expect. I know when to be close to a bathroom and when to tailor my activities as necessity permits. I thought I had the flare routine down as I had been through it so many times. Ha! I *thought* I had it down, but my colon was over *that* boring routine and gave me a surprise I will never forget…

I woke up around 5am on a crisp May morning. My husband and I had an hour-and-a-half drive ahead of us as he was racing in an omnium, which is three bicycle races over the course of two days. I excitedly got in the car for our morning journey, was chipper as can be, and was definitely ready to see my husband kick some ass. We were about an hour into the drive when my little sphincter decided it wanted some attention and started quivering. I remember thinking, Squeeze, squeeze, squeeze. Keep this turtle head in. Don't shit your pants. *Squeeze...squeeze...squeeze. Got to find a bathroom NOW!* The problem was, it was balls early and I wasn't sure if we were going to find a place. Luckily, a grocery store was open, so I ran in and let it flow. *Aaaahhh, instant relief.* I walked back to the car, got in, and drove off, not thinking too much into it as I wasn't flaring at the time, or so I thought.

When we were five minutes from our destination, my sphincter once again started quivering like it was rocking out at a twerking competition. This time, it was a bit more urgent and I knew I'd better find a bathroom fast or I was going to be stuck an hour and a half from home with a mess in my pants and no change of clothes. I clenched my butt cheeks together with superwoman might and prayed I would find a bathroom quick. I desperately spotted a tiny small-town diner open, so I jumped out of the car and ran inside. It was obvious I was not a small-town local as every single person turned around to stare at me as I rushed in. I ran up to the counter, looked the older woman at the register in the eye, and urgently said, "Do you have a bathroom I can use? I'll buy coffee or whatever you want me to on my way out." I could tell that she sensed the desperation in my voice as she pointed to a teeny-tiny bathroom with a thin wooden door right next to the kitchen. *Damn,* I thought, *I have to crap by the kitchen? That's messed up!* I quickly rushed into the bathroom, locked the door, and let it rip. *I know* the locals heard me tearing it up through the thin wooden door. *Damn, can I get a break?* I thought. I turned around, looked into the bowl and definitely saw 'rhea, but no blood. By this point, I was confused and wasn't quite sure what was going on with my colon and her BFF, the sphincter, as I had never had urgency issues with the absence of blood.

When I was done, I gathered my courage, took a deep breath, and walked out into the tiny diner. As I walked out, the customers gave me a standing ovation. Just kidding! But by their glances, I knew they had heard the grand performance I gave moments before. I walked up to the lady behind the counter, ordered a small tea and a muffin as promised, and walked out the front door. I was glad to have made it to the bathroom, but started getting nervous as I had no idea what was going on with my bowels.

The rest of the morning and early afternoon went along without my sphincter seeking another standing ovation worthy performance, or more eloquently put, going into uncontrollable spasms. I was relieved and thought that it had been some sort of freak thing that happened earlier that morning and had nothing to do with possibly flaring.

By late afternoon, I was waiting for my husband's last race to start, nonchalantly talking to a fellow race spectator about the days' races when, out of nowhere, *BAM!!!* My lower abdominals started cramping like it was their job, my sphincter started to contract like it was trying to win the spasm Olympics, and I was sure I was about to shit my pants right there. I instantly sprinted away to find a bathroom, leaving an extremely confused dude in my wake as I ran off, mid-conversation, with no explanation.

As I sprinted to find a bathroom, I tried to clench my butt cheeks together with all of my might. However, running and clenching just don't go together, and I was sure a poo accident was inevitable. Luckily, I found a bar, ran in, and without having to say anything to the bartender, she pointed me to the bathroom. My face must have told her all that she needed to know. Ladies and gents, I am proud to announce that is the moment where my "shit face" was born. I was able to communicate without saying, "Lady, I gotta shit, and if you don't tell me where your bathroom is right now, I'm going to shit in the spot your hostess greets people for dinner." Thank God for my "shit face" because I actually made it to the bathroom, against all odds. My sphincter finally couldn't take being suppressed any longer and started to release. I instantaneously slid my bum onto the commode and let the poo party begin. Thank goodness I slid onto home plate just in time, otherwise, well, I don't want to think about the otherwise part. Again, I didn't have a change of clothes with me, my cell phone was in the car, and my husband was racing at the time. I would have been screwed with a capital S if I hadn't made it!

By this point, I was dumbfounded. I had never experienced flare-like symptoms with the absence of blood and always had a buildup of symptoms before getting to the shitting-pants-is-imminent stage. It usually took two to three weeks after a standard flare to get to the uncontrollable bowel movement stage. There was, however, only one explanation for the poo madness. I was flaring. It truly sucked to have no idea that I was going to have a curious case of the shitties all day.

Scared, confused, and wrecked with anxiety, I decided to not eat or drink for the rest of the day. That was the *only way* to guarantee I would not possibly shit my pants. After my husband finished his last race of the day, we made the hour-and-a-half drive home, went to sleep, got up the next morning, and did it all over again. This time, I did not eat or drink anything for fear that if I did I would possibly have an accident. For the second day in a row, I forgot a change of clothes. I went the entire second day without my sphincter quivering or my butt cheeks clenching because

I did not eat or drink anything from the moment I awoke. Putting my body into starvation mode was *not* what I wanted to do, but it had to be done out of pure necessity.

After my husband completed the omnium, we ate close to home as there were no guarantees my bowels were going to play nice with food. I could feel my bowels awaken as I began to drink and eat for the first time since I awoke twelve hours prior. Within thirty minutes, I was urgently rushing to the bathroom. As I yet again rushed to the bathroom for the umpteenth time that weekend, I remember begrudgingly thinking, *Damnit! I'm flaring! Not again!*

I made an appointment with my gastroenterologist the next morning, hoping to God I would get over this sneaky shyster of a flare quickly. I was knocked off my game as this flare came in like a lion and there were no guarantees, like all the others, that it would go out like a lamb.

The main thing this particular flare taught me was to always plan for the unexpected, even when I thought I was in remission and healthy. I had *no idea* I was flaring that day and would have been caught high and dry, or wet and smelly, if I would have crapped my pants. I also learned to not dismiss any "out of the ordinary" symptoms because they didn't fit in with my normal "flare" type activity. So, moral of the story is to always have a change of clothes in your trunk and call your doc if shit hits the fan, or splatters the toilet in an unfamiliar way, to ensure your flare doesn't get out of control!

The relaxing summer I was banking on did not happen that year.

There would be no such thing as worry-free summer bliss for me. Nope. It was yet another time that the ruthless disease hijacked my body, ransacked and stripped each cell of nutrients, ripped hope out of my soul, and was literally on the verge of leaving me for dead. Not only was my body reduced to a skeleton, but my mind was also starting to truly break down.

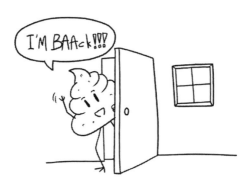

From July to early September, I rarely left the house as I could not control my bowels from unleashing "the beast," or more commonly known as bloody 'rhea, up to eighteen times a day. Even with no food in my system, my bowels would release a dark red substance that looked like oatmeal if I so much as drank a glass of water. It did not make sense to me. I was also starting to juggle a cocktail of drugs. I had built up antibodies to Remicade, which is why it was no longer working. So, in an attempt to help kick my body into remission, my gastroenterologist kept me on Remicade and Lialda, and added azathioprine and Entocort to my daily routine. I can't say I was happy about that, but the flare was severely taking a toll on my mind and body, so I was willing to try anything.

If I left the house, it was purely out of necessity to buy groceries, toiletries, or to see my gastroenterologist. On days I left the house, I did *not eat or drink anything* and made sure to carry a makeshift toilet made out of a paper grocery bag cut in half and stuffed with a plastic trash bag to ensure the leakage would not get all over the back of my car. Not eating or drinking was the only way to ensure I would not crap my pants in public. And that, my friends, was beginning to be more than I could handle. Driving around with a makeshift toilet helped ease my anxiety, but tugged at my soul. I never thought that at the age of twenty-eight I would yet again need to drive around with a freakin' paper bag toilet. More often than not, I would sob while driving around running errands as my uncontrollable bowels were starting to become too much to handle.

Month by month, I got sicker and sicker, skinnier and skinnier, more malnourished than ever. Not only was I on a heavy cocktail of drugs, but I was also eating the cleanest I ever had. It didn't matter how many meds I took or how clean I ate, none of it had an impact on my colon. It was getting to a point where no matter how positive I tried to be, my mind was breaking down. I felt as though the disease was not only starving my body, but starving my spirit. I also felt that the disease was starving the life out of me no matter how hard I tried to give it what it wanted.

I distinctly remember driving by the water, next to hundreds of beautiful evergreen trees with bald eagles carelessly flying through the blue sky, thinking that the disease was going to take my life that year. I told God that though I do not understand *why* I am going through this suffering, I fully surrender, have made my peace, and that I knew my time was near.

Everything I tried was failing. My diet was absolutely pristine. I tried things that promised to "cure," even against my better judgment. I was desperate to get better. No matter what. I would have done *anything* short of selling my soul to get better.

I will never forget walking into my gastroenterologist's office and *begging him to remove my colon.* I told him that I couldn't live like this anymore. I remember saying, "Doc, seriously, please remove my colon! You're pretty certain I have ulcerative colitis, right?! If we remove my colon, we remove the problem, right?!!"

"You don't want that, Emma," he replied. I remember being so pissed with his response! How dare he not want to remove my colon! I wanted to be normal so badly that I was willing to live with a colostomy bag for the rest of my life! At the time, I didn't care, and I remember being genuinely angry at him for rejecting my pleas to remove my colon, but instead of giving into my impulsive desires, he suggested the drug Cimzia. *Bullshit! I'm not trying another biologic drug!* I thought, *I'm over this!*

I was close to rock bottom when my husband came home from work on my birthday and told me to get dressed because he wanted to take me to dinner. I instantly panicked and told him I didn't want to go. He pleaded with me and told me that it would be good for me to get out of the house. I reluctantly agreed and prayed to God that I would make it to the bathroom if need be.

I jumped in the shower and when I got out, I caught a glimpse of myself in the mirror. I broke into sobs because I did not recognize the skeleton resemblance of somebody I once knew staring back at me. *What has happened to me?* I wondered in complete horror. I took a deep breath, gathered my emotions as best I could, and got dressed. We went to dinner and I spent my 29th birthday dinner picking at a piece of Alaskan salmon, taking teeny-tiny bites, wondering if this was going to be my last birthday celebration, and tried to put the fear of not making it to the restaurant bathroom in the back of my mind. I just wanted to be somewhat normal that evening. But again, scoping out bathrooms was my normal, and I had to try and just let any preconceived notions of normal go. It got me out of the house, and I appreciated the persistence of my husband to try and make my birthday as normal and nice as possible. I was happy I went, but was saddened by the anxiety that had become my norm. I just wanted a break. I wanted to not have to worry about bathrooms, or what the cocktail of meds was doing to my body, though it was apparent it wasn't helping sooth the ulcerations in my gut. I could have never predicted that a few weeks later, poo "accidents," bathroom emergencies, and drug cocktails would no longer seem like such a big deal.

On Labor Day weekend, my dad came to visit. The airport was an hour drive from our house, so my husband went to pick up my dad as it was obvious I would not be able to make the drive without experiencing severe anxiety about needing to get to a bathroom within seconds. After my husband returned home with my dad, my dad took one look at me and tried to play it off as if he wasn't deeply alarmed by my appearance. By this point, I had withered down to ninety-five pounds. At 5'1", my normal weight was somewhere between 115-120 pounds.

We didn't leave the house that weekend, but instead relaxed and did a bit of self-reflection. My dad told me that I needed to let go of the things that were eating me up. *What's eating me up?* I thought. I was somewhat clueless, but knew that, at some point during my journey, I'd figure it out.

While my dad was visiting, I was trying the fruitarian diet—my last-ditch effort to try and heal myself on my own. Everything that I tried up to that point had failed, and alarmed with my degrading condition, my gastroenterologist recommended that I go on Cimzia. I told him to pound sand and hoped to God that the fruitarian diet would provide me with some much-needed relief. My dad saw what I was doing and frankly stated, "You need to eat some food little girl." I meekly smiled and told him I would add a soup with more "substance." I decided to steam sweet potato with fresh celery juice, and when done, would blend the same steamed celery juice with the sweet potato to make a "soup" that I added into my diet (this soup was fruitarian approved). My flares hadn't experienced a drastic improvement, but I was experiencing a few formed bloody turds. That was a major victory in itself as I hadn't seen a formed turd in months! I was still extremely ill, but sometimes, the little victories make a big difference in psyche, even if it is short lived.

The evening my dad left, I made an organic tuna casserole and ate a little bit of it to show him that I was *trying* to eat something of substance. After dinner, my dad gave my fragile body a bear hug and headed off to the airport with my husband. I can guarantee you he was probably praying harder than he ever had in his life as he walked out the door that night.

As I was cleaning up, I felt as though I was being stabbed in the gut, my sphincter started quivering, and I sprinted to the bathroom. I made it to the toilet, but this particular bowel movement was different than any I had ever experienced.

Not only was I experiencing involuntary painful sphincter spasms, but my core body temperature dropped and I started shivering uncontrollably. I was definitely a little concerned, so I tried to think, *Mind over matter, mind over matter, stop shivering. No need to be shivering.* But mind over matter did not make a difference. I could not control the shivering. After what seemed like eternity, though it was only thirty minutes, I was able to remove myself from the toilet, clean myself up, and weakly stumble to the couch in extreme exhaustion. When my husband got home, he found me on the couch, covered in blankets, shivering. I explained to him what had happened and he encouraged me to go upstairs and take a hot shower.

After taking a hot shower, I crawled in bed beside my husband. I looked at him and said, half-jokingly, "When you wake up for work tomorrow, please make sure I'm alive." He told me to call my gastroenterologist first thing in the morning, and because we both mutually agreed that I was extremely ill, that I should probably pack an overnight hospital bag "just in case." I told my husband that I was ready for steroids, that's probably all I needed, and was "sure" I would be able to go home after seeing the doctor. I never, in a million years, was prepared for the reality check that happened the following day.

On September 7th, 2010, I learned just how fragile life is; to be exact, how fragile my life was. I called my gastroenterologist's office and explained the uncontrollable shivers that I experienced the night before. I was told to come in immediately. I gathered my hospital bag and favorite pillow just in case, though I was certain that I would not be admitted into the hospital. "I'll go on prednisone now. I'm sure that's all I need. I'll be back to normal in no time," I told my husband after finally agreeing that it was time to put my nine-month prednisone hiatus to bed.

I, of course, starved myself that morning as my gastroenterologist's office was an hour and a half away from where we lived. When we arrived in my gastroenterologist's office, I was put on the scale and weighed a whopping ninety-five pounds. *Damn, the fruitarian diet is no joke. I think the last time I was ninety-five pounds was in middle school,* I thought to myself, totally oblivious of the magnitude of my situation.

My gastroenterologist walked in, sat down, took one look at me, and sat back with his hand over his mouth. I could tell he was deep in thought as he intently stared at me. When he spoke, I was blown away with what he said.

"Emma, my first priority is to save you. My second priority is to save your colon."

Still not understanding the significance of what he was saying, I replied, "Doc, I'm totally ready to go on the prednisone now."

He then said, "Emma, you're going to be hospitalized for several weeks. Are you dizzy? We need to get you to the hospital right away."

Here I was, thinking I was going to be sent home with a shiny orange bottle of prednisone, but instead, I was going to be hospitalized for *several weeks?* I was surprised, but not too surprised.

The hospital was a block from my gastroenterologist's office, so I told him I would walk over. He was skeptical and wanted to send an ambulance for me, but I assured him that I would be fine. This was, yet again, another example of me not willing to accept how grave my condition truly was. My husband and I walked over to the hospital and I was admitted due to severe malnutrition and the continuous, severe bloody poo flare that I had experienced for the past nine months. I felt like this hospitalization was some sort of grand finale my colon had in store for me. Not thrilled to be in the hospital, I decided to roll with it and hope for the best.

After I was shown to my room, a PICC line was inserted and I was put on Total Parental Nutrition (TPN) and IV steroids known as Solu-

Medrol. The TPN was to feed my weakened, malnourished body while the Solu-Medrol would hopefully help the healing process in my colon. Once I was settled, the colorectal surgeon walked in. In a gentle voice, he said, "Emma, I'm the colorectal surgeon. There is a 50/50 chance we are going to have to remove your colon, but are hoping we won't have to because your body is too weak for surgery."

At that moment, I finally felt the weight of the situation. *Too weak for surgery? Like, I could die? Seriously? I can really die from ulcerative colitis? Oh, my gosh!* The irony was that a few months earlier I was begging my gastroenterologist to remove my colon so I could have quality of life, so I thought. It's incredible how the ball turned when I was faced with a 50/50 chance of major surgery and actually losing my colon. I was scared shitless. Well, I wouldn't say scared shitless because I was still shitting blood, *but* the true reality of living without a colon finally caught up to me. I was super sick. And I could possibly die. Damn. I know I spent all summer mentally preparing and trying to accept this situation, but nothing ever prepares you for actually facing it.

Two days later, I had a colonoscopy, and though my colon was severely diseased, it was starting to regenerate its tissues, cells, and skin. I was healing!!! *Hallelujah!!!* I was able to dodge the colon removal surgery, and after a week, was switched from IV steroids to oral steroids. Once my blood count stabilized, my protein levels were back to normal, and my colon showed that it could tolerate food, I was able to go home. But it was no walk in the park.

I was happy to be out of the hospital, but was in excruciating joint pain due to the quick steroid taper. I was thankful for it, but it was painful. For months after this hospitalization, I needed to get weekly massages to relieve the joint pain. Though my colon had healed in the hospital, it took my body months to recover and heal from the trauma it had experienced, relentlessly, for the past nine months.

Through this experience, I learned that life is a wonderful gift and I must be thankful for it every day. I was blessed to escape the hospital with my colon and was thrilled that my life was starting anew. It was a damn hard year, an emotional rollercoaster to be exact, but it was time to accept that for what it was and to keep pressing on. The road to recovery was not easy, but I learned to manage. I always tried to keep a positive attitude, keep the faith, and know that no matter what happened, I was alive and finally healthy again.

I was hospitalized three times the first four years after my ulcerative colitis diagnosis. This hospitalization was by far the most dangerous due to *severe* malnutrition and a flare that had gotten seriously out of control. This experience was an incredible learning moment and I now act when I experience symptoms instead of waiting to see what happens, or merely hoping that the disease will go away on its own. I've learned it definitely won't.

Though I have experienced many dark moments with this disease, I am thankful for the journey. It has taught me to live life to the fullest and to be thankful for each and every day on this earth. You, too, will figure out what works for you and your individual healing journey. I encourage you to rise with the sun every morning and know that you are here for a purpose, and that no matter how bleak moments may seem, they will get better. I am living proof as are so many others who have suffered from ulcerative colitis and Crohn's disease.

Whoa, Baby!!

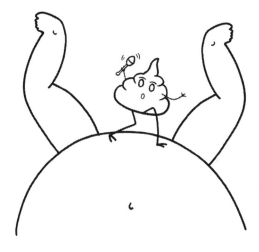

When my husband and I got married, I was a bit indifferent to having children. I was twenty-three when we married, and the last thing I wanted to think about was having a baby. At the time, we were both open to the idea of having children in the future but wanted to focus on building a life together and building a strong career foundation. I was diagnosed with ulcerative colitis ten months after we got married, and having kids was not even on my mind. After I became ill, experiencing flare after flare, our mindset shifted from being open to the idea of children, to indifference, to not even considering having a baby because we needed to focus our energy and efforts on keeping me healthy. The sicker I became, the more I was convinced that I would never be able to have children. I decided it was never possible for me to get pregnant due to the trauma my body suffered by repeated flares. I thought that the repeated flares coupled with years of never-ending medication cocktails pretty much sealed the deal for me. I had convinced myself that I would never have a baby, and I was okay with that. I told myself that I didn't like kids, that they were nasty "germ carrying rats" and that they would just get me sick all the time anyway due to my medicinally induced compromised immune system.

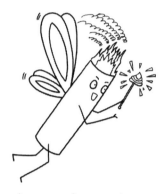

In June 2013, eight years after my ulcerative colitis diagnosis, my body went into a mild flare with the reappearance of the infamous bloody 'rhea and extreme cramping. It seemed that the lovely *flare fairy* hit me with her lightning bolt shit wand, deciding that it was time my asshole bolt out some 'rhea. My doctor put me on a short three-week low dose prednisone regimen, and I obliged after learning my lesson the hard way from the unforgettable 2010 hospitalization. I tapered off the prednisone and was confused when, after tapering, I still felt bloated and tired. My past experience told me that the prednisone side effects should have worn off. *What else could it be?* I thought. I was at a loss for what was going on, but didn't pay too much attention to it. Until I realized that my period was two weeks late. *Could I be pregnant? Could I be? Nah, I'm sure I'm not. My body is probably still thrown off from the 'roids,* I thought to myself. I decided I should take a pregnancy test "just in case," though my hubby insisted I was wasting money on a pregnancy test as he, too, thought my body was thrown off from the prednisone and had accepted the fact that we would probably never have kids.

I bought the pregnancy test, stopped at a local coffee shop on my way home, got home, and popped a squat on the commode, trying not to pee on my hand. I set the pregnancy test down, washed my hands, looked down at the test and did a double take! *WHAT THE WHAAAAT?!* Words cannot describe the absolute shock, excitement, and joyous emotional overload that I felt the moment I looked at the pregnancy test and realized I was pregnant! Hallelujah! This was *not* supposed to happen!! I was ecstatic and just knew, deep down, that everything was going to be fine. I instantly told all of my family and friends as a miracle had just happened! Not only was I pregnant, but my little baby survived in my womb though I was flaring shortly after she was conceived. I had no idea I was pregnant when I took the prednisone to calm my flare, and I was also on azathioprine and Lialda at the same time.

I was also wowed that I was *excited* to be pregnant. I had convinced myself that I didn't like children. How could I all of a sudden be absolutely elated? I then realized that perhaps my dislike for children was a protection mechanism because I never thought I would be able to have kids.

I informed my doctors right away that I was pregnant, and thus commenced the *medication wars* between my OB and my gastroenterologist. My OB wanted me to stop taking azathioprine and told me that if I flared again then they would treat me with prednisone, as that was a much safer drug for the baby inside my womb. My gastroenterologist assured me that he had several patients over the years who had been on azathioprine and their babies were perfectly fine. He was very firm with me when he stated that not taking the azathioprine and going into a severe flare would be much more dangerous for the baby then the azathioprine itself. Ultimately, I put my trust in my gastroenterologist and stayed on azathioprine while pregnant. I did, however, discontinue Lialda usage.

Prior to being pregnant, I had already struggled with being on immunosuppressant therapy, but now that I had another life to worry about I absolutely did not want to make the wrong decision. It was no longer about me. It was now all about my baby. I went back and forth several times, sometimes thinking I would stop the azathioprine completely, and at other times, thinking that I should trust in my gastroenterologist. He had saved my life and my colon in 2010, so I fully trusted him when it came to this matter. Ultimately, I decided to stay on 75mg of azathioprine throughout my pregnancy. Aside from the mild flare that I went through in the very beginning of my pregnancy (before I even knew I was pregnant), my body stayed in remission during my entire pregnancy.

It was amazing and I felt amazing! I felt as though my disease was cured and I would never have to worry about it again! I decided that I was going to have a natural birth, without the epidural, and hire a doula to assist my husband and I in the hospital. A natural birthing center or home birth led by a midwife was not an option for me and was completely out of the question due to my complicated medical history. To me, the risk to the baby was not worth any personal gain. Having been so sick in the past, I knew how quickly a normal situation could turn horrendous in a matter of seconds. I was not willing to take that chance with the most precious gift entrusted to me by God. I decided the next best thing was having a natural birth in the hospital without the epidural. I thought to myself, *How bad can it really be? I've suffered severe cramping while flaring, I've got this!* At least, so I thought!

A week before my daughter's original due date, I came down with a cold accompanied by a mild fever and cough. I decided that I wanted my immune system to be as strong as possible for the delivery of my daughter so I stopped taking azathioprine. I blamed my fever and cold on the immunosuppressant azathioprine, and because I had done great during my pregnancy, I was confident in my decision to stop the drug. My daughter decided not to arrive on her original due date, but that was of no concern to me because I felt it gave my body enough time to completely get the medication out of my system.

My daughter was two weeks late, so my OB decided she was going to induce me. Two days before I was supposed to be induced, I started feeling intense cramping. I actually thought I was in labor because the pain was so intense, but knew it was not true labor, so I laid in bed and sucked it up. Staying true to the warrior spirit my daughter possessed from conception, I went into labor twelve hours before I was supposed to get induced. I remember taking literally four hours to try and eat and shower before my husband drove me to the hospital. I was SO miserable from labor pains! Freaking balls, it was the most intense thing I've ever felt! I abandoned the non-epidural option and decided to get the epidural, as I hadn't really slept for forty-eight hours prior to going into labor.

My water still hadn't broken, so my OB came in to break my water. As she broke my water, she noticed poo, or meconium, was present. She said I should be fine, and that they'd monitor the baby and myself during delivery. When it was time to push, I gave it all I had. I pushed like it was my job, and I shat on the table several times while pushing! Trust me when I say that crapping on the table in front of your labor nurse or OB doc is NO BIG DEAL after dealing with Crohn's disease or ulcerative colitis!

I ended up developing a fever while in labor, and slowly, my contractions started to stop. The baby was in distress, and with my fever, things did not look bright. It turned out that my daughter was stuck, I was in distress because of my fever, and things could turn really bad real fast. We ultimately decided an emergency cesarean was a much better choice than trying to force my daughter out via vacuum, and thank goodness we chose that option. When my daughter was delivered, it took her a little while to take her first breath. My husband, being the stoic man that he is, didn't alert me that anything was wrong. I asked him, "Is the baby out yet?"

"Yes." He replied in a calm, cool manner.

"Why isn't she crying?" I asked.

"They're waking her up." He said. At the time, I didn't think anything of it, but what I didn't realize was that the baby didn't wake up right away and took a little while to breathe. But, when she was ready, she took her first breath. And screamed. Covered in poo. Yes, yes, this is MY daughter! She made her grand entrance by waking up when *she* wanted to and then screamed, in all her glory, covered in poo. Glorious, simply glorious.

I was able to briefly look at my daughter before she was taken away by a team of doctors, my husband in tow, to get her lungs checked, as they did not know if she had inhaled the meconium into her lungs. I was left alone with the delivery team sewing me up and the anesthesiologist caressing my head.

I woke up three hours later in a foreign hospital room, alone. I sat up, confused, wondering where everybody was. I did not have my phone with me and had no idea what was going on with the baby. I didn't feel as though I had just had a baby. It didn't go at all the way I'd envisioned. Instead of having my daughter suckle on my breast the moment after I delivered her, I was alone in a hospital room. So many thoughts were racing through my mind and I couldn't help but wonder if I was going to be one of *those women* who simply couldn't bond with their child. Laying alone in the hospital bed of a room I didn't recognize, staring blankly at the clock on the wall directly in front of me, with an empty womb, my thoughts started creeping to the dark side. *What if I don't love my baby? What if I don't like being a mom? Where is my baby? Where is my husband? Why don't I feel like I just had a baby? Why don't I feel anything at all? Why don't I have any emotion right now? What is going on with me?*

About that moment, my husband rushed into the room. I asked him where the baby was and wanted to know what the heck was going on because I was completely clueless. He told me our daughter had to be hooked up to an IV, an oxygen tube, monitoring equipment, and had to reside in the "nursery" until she was properly treated for any possible infection resulting from the meconium exposure.

Once I could move my legs, they allowed me to go into the nursery to breastfeed my baby. Almost six hours after she was born, I took her tiny body into my arms and instantly felt all of the emotions and feelings *I should have felt* the moment I gave birth to her. Overwhelming unconditional love flooded every inch of my being. I couldn't believe it. I was finally a mom.

Luckily, my daughter, Gisele, never got sick from the meconium. We were able to leave the hospital three days after I delivered her. She took to the breast right away and was breastfeeding like a champ. I felt good, my poo looked great, and other than the pesky cesarean section, I felt amazing! My daughter was a healthy eight pounds and would definitely continue to chunk up with the way she was eating. The first two weeks postpartum, I continued to feel great. I felt like I was glowing and still felt healthy. Deep down, I hoped that the disease would stay in remission for eternity, but that sort of dreamy postpartum flare-free life I envisioned definitely would not happen for me.

Three weeks after my daughter was born, I began flaring. Within a week, the flare had me running to the bathroom several times a day, releasing bloody poo. I was concerned about my milk supply and refused to become malnourished and sick with a newborn. My baby *would not* sit in a rocker in the bathroom as I released bloody stool into the commode. Hell no, I wasn't having that mess…literally! I know mother-baby bonding is important, but *come on,* not at *that* level!

I called my gastroenterologist and asked for a Hydrocortisone enema as that had helped calm flares in the past and put me in remission without the need for prednisone. The Hydrocortisone enema was prescribed, but did little to nothing to calm the symptoms of this quickly approaching out of control flare. After the shock of the enema failing to work, I realized that I had only one option. Prednisone. I was not willing to risk my milk supply nor toss my baby in her rocker just so I could avoid my prednisone nemesis. No, no, NO!

I immediately called my gastroenterologist and asked to be put on prednisone. I was asked to wait two weeks as I originally had a colonoscopy scheduled, and the gastro doc couldn't scope me earlier because he was going on vacation. Um, yeah, I definitely refused that one. *Sorry, doc, my colon doesn't go on vacay from exploding bloody shit just because you're on vacation!*

My doctor's office, understanding my unique circumstances, agreed and put me on prednisone. To my horror, prednisone did not work right away. I started freaking out, thinking that maybe I had colon cancer and that's why the prednisone wasn't kicking my body into remission. So many thoughts I never knew I could possess passed through my mind. At that moment, all I wanted, more than anything, was to see my daughter grow up. I was absolutely terrified! It was no longer just my husband, my flare and I, but was now my husband, myself and our daughter, with no room for flaring. It took two weeks being on prednisone to kick my body into remission, but it finally started working.

The weeks leading up to my colonoscopy seemed to drag on forever. I just wanted to ensure I didn't have colon cancer. I wanted the comfort of knowing it was just a flare due to the stress of being a new mom and the wonderfully shocking miracle my body went through to birth my daughter. The new thoughts that went through my mind blew me away. The last thing a new mom wants to do is go on a medication that will blow her up like a freakin' hot air balloon! But I did. I begged for the prednisone because it was no longer about me. It was about being an effective mom and making the most nourishing milk for my daughter.

My colonoscopy came and went and revealed that my colon did show signs of active disease but showed zero signs of colon cancer. I was finally able to breathe easy. My gastroenterologist told me that he was going to do a slow taper of the prednisone over the course of five months. Normally, I would freak out, but not this time. With the scare of the flare symptoms, I decided to restart 75mg of azathioprine and Lialda. I simply waited four hours after taking the azathioprine to breastfeed my daughter as an "above and beyond" precaution. But I'm here to tell you, when it comes to the health of your child, there is no such thing as an "above and beyond" precaution.

It was hard being on prednisone when I was trying to lose baby weight, but that was not nearly as important as being healthy for my daughter, not having mommy-baby bonding sessions over the commode, and me being able to produce and feed her breast milk as long as I could. The prednisone-induced hot air balloon silhouette I touted around had nothing on any of that! I will forever be thankful for my body's amazing ability to produce breast milk despite the persistent flare symptoms and the continued use of potent medications. My breast milk never dried up and I was able to nourish my daughter until it was time to wean her off, which was well after her first birthday.

It took me a little over two years to lose my "prednisone baby weight." At the end of my five-month stint with prednisone coupled with an inconsistent diet, I was heavier than I was two weeks after giving birth to my daughter. With the stress and lack of sleep of being a new mom, moving from the West coast to East coast when my daughter was six months old, trying to hold down the home front, and not eating as well and as disciplined as I had in the past, it seemed like I could not release the weight. But I was healthy and my daughter was healthy. I had to remind myself frequently that being healthy was what was most important, as it was hard to look in the mirror and see an overweight version of a woman I once knew.

In January of 2016, I got pregnant with my second child. Unfortunately, at the six-week mark, I miscarried. This proved to be challenging emotionally, but I never experienced flare-like symptoms during my short pregnancy or after. There was never any evidence that inflammatory bowel disease had anything to do with the miscarriage we suffered, however, we will never know for sure.

In May of 2016, I had a sneaking suspicion that I was pregnant because my turds quickly turned from average to five-star overnight. Like, seriously, if there was a turd competition, I would win gold! I remember looking into the toilet and thinking to myself, *Damn, that beaut came out of me?! There must be something going on!! I must be pregnant or something.* Sure enough, I took an early pregnancy test and it came out positive. Whoa-whoa-wee-wow! I was pregnant!! I thought for sure I would sail through the pregnancy with minimal issues in the colon department as I had done so well while pregnant with Gisele. With these five-star turds building up my confidence, I thought I was bulletproof. Alas, I couldn't have been more wrong.

I started having minor flare-like symptoms at week five of my pregnancy. My farts and poo started smelling like the all too familiar and all too eerie good ol' flare "open wound" smell. That bitch of a flare fairy had definitely paid my colon a visit. *Damnit!* I thought. Trying to get out ahead of this thing, I called my gastro doc and asked for the Hydrocortisone enema. I had stopped Lialda but was still on 50mg of azathioprine. They prescribed the enema and asked for a shit load of stool samples to see what was going on inside that pesky little colon of mine. The *last thing* I ever wanted to do whilst pregnant, and with the beginning stages of pregnancy morning sickness nausea, is shit into a container, sift through my bloody shit to put into lab containers, and take it to the lab. My pregnancy nose was on par with that of a bloodhound, so this *shit and sift session* was definitely brutal, even with me wearing a mask. I remember being relieved when it was over, but disheartened by the blood in my poo. I kept the faith, believing that this was going to be a very minor flare and that the Hydrocortisone enema would stop this flare pronto.

I started the Hydrocortisone enema and, though I experienced "manageable" symptoms, my colon was not healing as quickly as I would have liked. After two weeks of Hydrocortisone enema use, my gastroenterologist recommended that I also add in a Canasa suppository daily. My asshole TLC regimen consisted of a Canasa suppository in the morning and Hydrocortisone enema in the evening. Again, as a pregnant woman, the *last thing* I wanted to do was stick stuff up my arse first thing in the morning and last thing at night. However, what I did and did not want to do was no longer a luxury afforded to me. I had to do what I needed to do to keep myself healthy so the little human growing within my belly could thrive.

I'm here to tell you, Hydrocortisone enemas while pregnant are most uncomfortable. Not only did I already feel bloated, but it compounded that feeling every time I injected the watery enema into my arse, leaving me feeling crampy and sick. Eight weeks into my pregnancy and two days after adding the Canasa suppository to my regimen, I noticed a remarkable improvement in my symptoms. The blood in my stool was slowly decreasing, the awful "sick" shit smell was dissipating, and I was beginning to see little turdlets resembling shrimp hanging out at the bottom of the toilet bowl after I shat. I felt confident that the worst was over and that I was finally on the mend. Again, I couldn't have been more wrong.

At week nine of my pregnancy, I was crapping straight 'rhea eight to ten times a day, and the bleeding had come back with a vengeance. By week ten, my colon smelled like there was a dead animal rotting in my gut. It was, by far, the foulest smell that had ever come out of my colon. The farts and poo that came out of my gut would clear a room in an instant as the smell was in a category of its own, inhuman of sorts. Aside from my postpartum flare, this flare was quickly becoming one of the most challenging of my life as there was absolutely no predictability to it. I was scared. I was worried about the tiny human growing inside my belly. How could this little being survive the harsh symptoms I was going through? The intense abdominal cramping, frequent blood loss from crapping eight to ten times a day, and my inability to eat or drink was brutal, disheartening, depressing, and scared the living shit out of me because I had no idea what was going on with my body.

It was clear the azathioprine was not helping, and I was quickly running out of options. I immediately contacted my gastroenterologist and asked for prednisone, and it was at that moment my entire world was rocked. My gastroenterologist agreed that prednisone was necessary to get a grip of the flare, but she also strongly encouraged me to consider going on Humira. *What the what?!! Humira…a biologic drug? START IT while pregnant?* Honestly, I thought my doctor was straight crazy. *Why would she recommend such a radical, drastic treatment?* I thought to myself. Up to this point, I had been off of biologics for six years, ranging from September 2010-September 2016. Prior to this pregnancy, I was almost off all of my medication. I had slowly tapered myself off of azathioprine, being at 50mg, well below the therapeutic dose for my height and weight.

I was crushed. I was so close, yet so far away from my medication freedom. I felt that my immune system wasn't too compromised for the past few years because I was on such a low dose of azathioprine. Now, all of a sudden, she is suggesting Humira? I was having serious issues accepting this fact. I politely told her I would prefer to try the 'roids, and if they didn't work, then I would *consider* going on Humira, though, deep down, I felt there was no way I was going on that drug, especially while pregnant. I felt that prednisone had to be the safest bet, so I just accepted the fact that I may potentially rival Shamu in appearance if stuck on prednisone for the majority of my pregnancy.

I thought prednisone was the safest option until I met resistance from my gastroenterologist on the matter. It wasn't until I spoke with her secretary that I realized *my gastroenterologist* was not only a subject matter expert in the area of medications used to treat IBD and pregnancy, but that she was also a researcher, having studied over 1,134,964 pregnant women over the course of two years to see which medications were safest between steroids, thiopurines, and anti-tumor necrosis factor (biologic) drugs (infliximab, adalimumab and certolizumab). Of these pregnant women, over 20,000 were exposed to these three particular medications. The study found that the use of anti-TNFs, or thiopurines, was found to be safe and not associated with an increased risk of poor outcomes like intrauterine growth retardation, stillbirth, or puerperal infection. The study did find that combination therapy of an anti-TNF drug and thiopurines was associated with an increased risk of preterm births and the risk for severe acute respiratory infection in the first two years of life.

I was shocked to discover that the use of steroids for women suffering from inflammatory bowel disease showed a significant increased risk for preterm birth, intrauterine growth retardation, and stillbirth. The study did note that it is possible that the side effects were not necessarily from the steroids themselves but from ongoing inflammation in the digestive tract that was masked by the steroids. It amazed me to find out that corticosteroids do not represent a safe treatment option.

What absolutely knocked my socks off was the study's conclusion. It concluded that the use of biologics and thiopurines in an IBD pregnancy is NOT associated with a higher risk of complications when compared with the general population, unless when used in combination with steroids. The study also stated that corticosteroids may be useful in an acute setting to control a flare-up, but long-term use in pregnancy is associated with poor outcomes for the mother and baby.[1]

After reading this study, by mind was blown. But, at the same

---

[1] Truta, Brindusa. "Potential Risks of Immunosuppressant Drugs to the Pregnant Patient." American College of Gastroenterology. 7 October 2015.

time, I was feeling incredibly blessed because *my gastro doc* was the study's author. It was at that moment that I realized what I thought I knew about meds, I didn't, and that it was time, for the first time in my life, to 100% trust my doctor when it came to the absolute right medication for my out of control colitis flare. Even if it included going on Humira. Freaking balls, it was hard to accept the fact that the best thing for me and my unborn baby was to go on a biologic drug. I had felt so successful being off of biologics for six years. I was proud of myself and my life choices for keeping me off of this potent medication. I appreciated not having a medication-induced compromised immune system. I was *so close* to coming off of all meds. And now, in the blink of an eye, I was having to go on Humira, a biologic drug. I knew it had to be done and was, ultimately, the right decision. I knew that I didn't have a choice because the health of me and my unborn baby depended on it.

Had I not been pregnant, I would have tried a twenty-eight day juice feast, drank lots of bone broth, meditated, and rested plenty. However, being pregnant, I *did not* have the luxury of experimentation as I did during previous flares. I was unwilling to put my unborn baby at risk. To add to that, my quality of life was marginal. Due to being severely ill, I did not leave my house from weeks eight to twelve of my pregnancy, with the exception of medical and lab appointments that were necessities. I could no longer take my two-year-old daughter to the park or out to play because I was simply too sick, too weak, and too afraid of shitting my pants in public. It was not the life that I'd envisioned. In what seemed like a blink of an eye, I had quickly gone from a vibrant, healthy, always on-the-go mom to a woman just hanging on by a thread, hoping that my unborn baby could hang on through the flare. At the same time, I felt extremely guilty for putting my daughter in front of the television to keep her occupied when I was too weak to get up from the couch, with the exception of sprinting to the commode when the lower abdominal cramping started. It was brutal and the ultimate mind fuck. It was extremely hard for me to accept the situation, but I had no choice. It was what it was, and I reminded myself that we, as a family unit, would get through this.

Desperate for a *functioning* and *normal* quality of life, I accepted the situation for what it was. I reminded myself of my long-term mantra of, "Just because you need a potent medication now doesn't mean you will need it forever," that I have often told others suffering from IBD. Taking a deep breath, I emailed my doctor and told her that I was ready to go on Humira.

I just wanted to be well. I wanted to take my daughter to the park, and I desperately wanted my unborn baby to be healthy. I started on 40mg of prednisone at week thirteen of my pregnancy and Humira at week fourteen of my pregnancy. I was a little worried about the combination therapy, but I also knew I did not have a choice because the flare was so out of control. My doctor would have preferred for me to also stay on azathioprine, but I politely declined.

I went into remission about four days after starting prednisone, which also happened to be my 35th birthday. It was also on that day that I had my second ultrasound. Much to the relief of my husband and I, our baby was thriving! Our little unborn baby was jumping, kicking, and dancing in utero! *Hallelujah, our baby's alive!* I thought, exhaling all anxiety and emotional turmoil. Thankfully, the flare did not take its toll on our little baby! I think it's safe to say that the outcome of that ultrasound was easily the best birthday gift I've ever received.

As I'm writing this book, I am currently still pregnant, but I have faith that our little one will be healthy and strong, regardless of the medication that I am on to control the disease. The most important aspect that this particular experience taught me is that sometimes there truly is no rhyme or reason to flare-ups. I suspect this flare was caused by the hormonal changes of pregnancy, but I can never say with certainty. Perhaps it was the cycle of the disease deciding that it wanted to attack my colon and wreak havoc on my life. I'll never know for sure. But what I do know is that only I could control how I was mentally affected by the flare-up. Though it was rocky at first, I pulled myself off the floor and reminded myself that I would get better.

The best advice I can give about having a baby is to talk with your doctor to make sure your body is healthy enough to carry and deliver a baby, and to make sure it is safe with the medication, if any, that you are taking. There are some medications used to treat IBD that one should not get pregnant or try to impregnate their significant other with while on. If your doctor gives you the green light and you want to have a baby, then DO IT (literally)! Family and friends may give you their opinions, either encouraging or discouraging, but don't let it affect you either way. Though it may be frustrating, take it all with a grain of salt and do what you feel deep in your heart is right. My mom was terrified that I was going to die during child birth, and I was actually nervous to tell her each time I got pregnant, but once she found out, she handled it well and was ecstatic.

I want to encourage you to never, ever lose hope. I never thought I would get pregnant due to the severity of my illness and endless drug cocktails. The fear of what a pregnancy may do to my body forced my husband and I to use protection more often than not. After we convinced ourselves that it was physically impossible for my body to get pregnant, we dropped the condoms, and a little after two years, we got pregnant! I never in a million years thought I would get pregnant, but it happened! If you want to have a baby, be patient with your body, don't stress about it, and most importantly, keep the faith! If it is meant to be, it will happen. What's most important is that you don't stress or obsess over it! Godspeed my fellow baby carriers and baby makers!!

Food: The Ultimate Crap Shoot

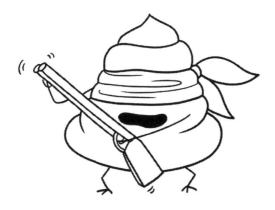

In the previous chapters, I've shared some of the good, the bad, and the ugly parts of my life with inflammatory bowel disease. While those amazing tales were unfolding, there was a parallel story taking place in the background. My struggle was not only with poo and the embarrassing situations my colon put me in, but I was also in a constant battle to find out what foods actually worked for my body. In the next few pages, I document the struggles that I have dealt with trying to find the "miracle diet" to cure myself of IBD. This food fight has been excruciating and is still, to this day, part of my ongoing IBD journey.

I never thought about what I put into my body prior to my ulcerative colitis diagnosis. I mean, *who does that* when you feel invincible and on top of the world?! After graduating from college, I lived on a steady diet of takeout, Mexican, and fast food. It was quick, easy, and greasily delicious, not to mention, super convenient. As a young professional, the last thing I wanted to burden myself with was the inconvenience of cooking! I was blessed with natural athletic ability and a skinny physique, so, yeah, why wouldn't I eat whatever I wanted? Food had no impact on me...or so I thought.

Immediately after my ulcerative colitis diagnosis, I still didn't understand the correlation that what you eat equals what will or will not wreck your colon. I was not educated at the time that food plays a *major factor* when it comes to healing your gut. Instead of mentioning dietary changes and planting the seed that I should perhaps change my diet, my gastroenterologist, at the time of my official diagnosis, instead sent me home with bright shiny pics of my severely ulcerated colon, a bottle of prednisone, and told me to come back in six weeks.

Almost every single time I ate "heavy" type foods such as red meat, dairy products, fast food, fried food, or drank beverages like soda or alcohol, I, or better yet, my colon almost always paid for it. I distinctly remember sitting on the commode with warm blood coming out of my arse thinking, *The food (or drink) did this to me. The food is making my condition worse. Oh, my gosh, there has got to be another way!* You would think that warm blood coming out of my arse would keep me from eating "naughty" foods, but no, it didn't. I had formed a bad habit, and it was one that I would not immediately conquer.

It was then that I realized I needed to self-educate myself about food and diet, and I better do it fast. I bought every book explaining the ins and outs of inflammatory bowel disease as well as books about food and "miracle" diets that swore if you followed their particular diet to the letter then you would eventually experience miraculous healing from all symptoms or long-term remission. *Yes, yes, this is what I need!* I thought. I was willing to do and try anything to heal my gut. Eighteen to twenty bloody 'rhea episodes a day convinced me it was time to try and find a healthy alternative to all the fried food debauchery that I had overindulged in.

The more books I read, the more hopeful I became (minus the scientific books on inflammatory bowel disease—they were downright boring and depressing). I slowly ditched the "doom and gloom" scientific literature on IBD and started reading more diet healing books. The first diet healing book I read was *The Maker's Diet* by Jordan Rubin. This book was quite revolutionary for me as I had absolutely *no idea* that the food I had been consuming for years was, well, subpar compared to what I should have been eating. I mean, come on, at twenty-four, why would I even know that farm raised salmon is way less nutritious, swims in its own shit, eats its own shit, and eats other dead farm raised salmon that, you guessed it, eats their own shit!! Seriously, if you are what you eat, I don't want to eat *that!* I already had enough of my own shit problems to worry about! I learned that wild caught salmon was much more delicious, nutritious, and extremely healthy for you! It blew my mind! Watch out Titanic, that was just the tip of the Iceberg.

The more revolutionary things I learned by reading *The Maker's Diet,* the hungrier for nutritional knowledge I became. Unable to put this book down, I learned the importance of organic meats and eggs. I learned to ditch cow products for goat products. What the what?! *There's such a thing as goat yogurt, cheese, and kefir?!* It sounds so silly to me now, over ten years later, but why would I *ever* think to consume products from a goat in my early twenties?! I didn't even know goats freaking lactated! Again, my mind was blown!

I quickly switched to organic meats, eggs, and goat products. *This was it!* I thought. I was *finally* going to experience health and long-term remission! Until I didn't.

Despite following *The Maker's Diet* quite religiously for several months, I still experienced flare after flare. I definitely felt much more empowered about my food choices because I was trying to take my health into my own hands and was making much better nutritional choices, but I could not understand why I did not experience the healing and long lasting remission that Jordan Rubin did. *What am I doing wrong?* I thought. *What is wrong with me? Is my colon just that far gone?*

Feeling a bit defeated, I decided to once again become a fast food crack junky. My husband, alarmed that I was starting down the never-ending deep, dark fast food hole once again, became more vocal and tried to tell me that enough was enough as gently as possible. Being the stubborn, hard-headed twenty-something that I was, I decided that I needed to go *Code Red*: Eat the junk food and then hide the carnage so he would never see it. I would go to fast food places, scarf down the food in my car, and then dump the evidence in the dumpster. He'd surely never realize this, right?

If alarm bells are going off in your head right now, you are ages ahead of where I was at that time in my life. It didn't dawn on me at the time, but I had begun a very dangerous cycle. I got temporary joy out of the super unhealthy fast food, but then was super sick in the form of bloody 'rhea and severe abdominal cramping shortly thereafter. But I kept doing it. At the time, I didn't realize why I was self-destructing. I knew what I *should do,* so why couldn't I just do it?

I couldn't do it because what I put into my mouth was *the only thing I could control* in my life. I felt that the newly healthy organic foods that I had switched too suddenly, and had put so much hope and faith in, had let me down when I couldn't stay in remission. So why shouldn't I eat what I wanted? It was all going to come out the same way anyhow. I liked the feeling of being able to control what I ate, and what I wanted to eat was out of control for my colon.

If there is anything a sick colon will do, it will eventually force you to pull your head out of the sand and change your life. Finally, after drinking a huge Dr. Pepper, I got super sick. Not just bloody 'rhea sick. I was nauseous, dizzy, and felt as though I was going to collapse. It was at that moment that I gave up soda for good, flipped the bird to fast food, and committed 100% to eating a healthy lifestyle.

My hunger for healthy food knowledge was reinvigorated and I was finally ready to commit 100% to changing my life for the better. As if God was speaking directly to me, I remember watching *The Tyra Banks Show* and seeing Alissa Cohen on set speaking about raw foods. I was blown away. I had never, not once, even considered eating only raw foods, which consist of only raw fruits and vegetables and sprouted or raw nuts, seeds, and legumes. Of these foods, none can be heated above 118 degrees. I instantly bought her book, dove in head first, and was wowed by what I read! Surely, this would be the miraculous healing that I needed!

With new-found motivation and feeling full of nothing but hope, I bought a juicer and was wowed by the blunt force and power that this new machine ripped vegetables and fruits apart with, producing a nutrient dense elixir that my body was so desperate for. This freshly made juice allowed me to absorb the nutrients of the fresh vegetable and fruit juices, which, in turn, helped me feel like Superwoman, yet not have the side effects of the fiber, because my ulcerated colon simply could not handle fiber at the time. It was a refreshing, healing way to get nutrition, which was something I had never given a second thought to in the past.

I slowly incorporated more and more raw foods into my diet and also continued to eat organic meat and goat products. I drank detoxification clay in distilled water daily. For the first time in my life, I started practicing yoga. It was time to finally heal. Except, again, after living this lifestyle for months, I didn't heal. I continued to flare on and off and was so frustrated with my lack of success in the remission department. *What am I doing wrong? Why can everybody else and their mama experience remission according to these miraculous diet books, but for some reason, I can't?* It was a mystery to me and left me extremely frustrated. But this time, I didn't give up nutritionally. I continued to have faith that I would heal, and that these new foods would be my answer.

Miraculously, the day after Thanksgiving of 2008, which was also right after my Remicade dosage was doubled, my body went into long-term remission. I didn't know it at the time, but I would experience remission for thirteen months. It was amazing. I had been off soda and fast food for almost a year up to that point. During this time, I continued to educate myself with health and wellness and nutrition books, and continued practicing yoga as well as riding my bike. As my remission continued, I slowly got bolder and bolder and would eat things I normally wouldn't eat, like seafood au-gratin with enough cream and dairy nastiness to wreck anybody's gut. I started consuming cow cheese like it was my job, eating cow ice cream and eating pizza. My discipline was starting to slip, though I always stayed true to a few of my core principles, which were no soda and no fast food, *no matter what.* There were no exceptions to this rule. I remember one night *not* eating because I flew into Florida on a late-night flight and the only thing open at the time was fast food "restaurants." I went hungry that night, as I would not compromise on my core principles.

In December of 2009, I started having light flare symptoms. You know the type, the smell of a dead animal rotting in your colon every time you poop or fart, diarrhea, and blood in the toilet. *Oh, no,* I thought. *It's happening again.* It was time to get disciplined, and that is exactly what I did. I felt a strong calling to revisit the raw foods lifestyle, so I joined an online raw foods support group and jumped right in. I refused to go into a full-blown flare. Surely, a raw diet, revisited, would be my answer. At the time, I felt that my colon was strong enough to handle going 100% raw, so that's what I did.

I felt so happy and free eating only raw foods. I mean, seriously, eating only organic fruits, vegetables, sprouted nuts, seeds, and legumes was so full of living nutrition and enzymes that I felt on top of the world. I felt so energetic! I was convinced that I would fully heal and be completely medicine-free! Heck, I didn't even look at it as a diet anymore. I looked at it as a lifestyle. *My lifestyle.* I felt like I was floating on clouds, nothing could stop me; I was finally going to conquer this disease!!

Until, that is, I fell through the clouds into a thunderstorm and got struck by lightning. I learned really fast that when flaring, a gourmet raw meal is not the ideal thing to eat. I ate everything from raw pizza to raw lasagna. All this raw goodness also made my butthole raw, as my colon simply could not handle the roughage!! Realizing that my miraculous raw foods lifestyle simply would not heal my colon, I decided to try the Specific Carbohydrate Diet (SCD). After a few months on this diet, I could no longer continue because, for some reason, the different foods and recipes of this particular diet started to repulse me. I simply could no longer bring myself to cook and eat anything that was recommended on SCD. I had never been so repulsed by a particular diet before, so thought it best to listen to my body telling me no, no, and NO! I ditched the SCD book, ditched the diet, and decided to form my own eating plan.

Yet again, I revisited the raw foods lifestyle, but instead, decided to eat more simple raw foods versus gourmet raw foods. In the morning, I would have a delicious smoothie, would have juice and a big heaping salad for lunch, and would eat some type of animal carcass like wild Alaskan salmon or organic chicken and veggies for dinner. This became my normal diet routine, and though this lifestyle did not completely put my body into remission, I felt that it did help to keep the mild ongoing flare that I was experiencing from moving to completely out of control.

Unfortunately, all bets were off when I got food poisoning from an undercooked piece of organic chicken in May of 2010. That undercooked piece of chicken awoke the beast in my gut and I began flaring out of control, complete with not being able to control my bowels, having bloody 'rhea roughly twenty times a day, and extreme abdominal cramping.

By the time my gastroenterologist tested me for E.coli, there was none present in my gut, which led me to believe that the organic chicken came, infected my colon with whatever nasty bacteria it contained, awakened the ulcer monsters in my colon, and then left. I seriously felt that the undercooked piece of carcass called the flare fairy and put a hit out on my colon! Not cool! To this day, I am extremely finicky when it comes to chicken and will inspect each piece before I eat it. And if it's not organic or raised by a farmer I trust, forget it! I won't touch it! Life's seriously too short for the game of chicken roulette!

My gastroenterologist pushed prednisone, but I refused because there was one diet I had not yet tried and I knew this one *had to be the answer!* It was the *fruitarian* diet.

Saddened and desperate to heal, I searched out a man named David Klein who said he'd cured himself of advanced ulcerative colitis by using natural hygiene and by eating only a raw foods diet. He is a huge advocate for the fruitarian diet. Fruitarians, as the name suggests, eat about 75% raw fruits, with the other 25% being raw vegan type foods. He encourages all of his clients suffering from IBD to try the fruitarian raw vegan diet and claims that he has a 99% success rate. Desperate for healing, I worked with him directly. I was extremely ill when I hired him in 2010, and during our first Skype session, he looked at me and told me I should be healed within two weeks. *Wow, is it really that easy? That would be a miracle!* I thought. I had suffered for four years with severe flare ups and was willing to try *anything*. Against my better judgment, I stopped taking all of my medications and embarked head first into the fruitarian lifestyle and also practiced natural hygiene.

After trying the fruitarian diet for three days, I had a formed bowel movement, which was the first formed log I had seen at the bottom of the toilet bowl in months! This beauty of a log was definitely promising, though it was still covered in blood, and despite this small success, I was still crapping eighteen to twenty times a day. A few days later, of those bowel movements, maybe two or three were formed. I felt myself growing sicker, weaker, thinner and more malnourished, but I held onto hope and continued to work with David directly. A few weeks later, I ended up in the hospital because my condition had deteriorated to a point where I almost didn't survive.

I don't blame David or the fruitarian diet for my quick and rapid decline as my colon was *so far gone* that I don't think anything but modern medicine could've brought my corpse-like body back to life. I do, however, have issues with him claiming that I would be healed in two weeks, and that he has a 99% success rate. To that, I raise a glass and say, *bullshit.* However, I think it is important for *every individual* suffering from IBD to try what path calls to them. The fruitarian diet called to me as a last resort, against my better judgment, and it didn't work. I tried it for less than a month, but again, my colon was so sick I truly believe nothing but modern medicine would have helped at that point. And that's okay. Just because it didn't work for me does not mean it won't work for you. We are all built and made differently.

After the infamous hospitalization in September of 2010, I was still unwilling to give up on the raw diet concept, so I read more books, sought out the experts in the field, and educated myself on *both* the pros and cons of the raw diet. In September of 2011, I met my raw foods idol, Alissa Cohen, and became a certified raw foods teacher under her *Living on Live Food* teacher certification program. I was determined to make the raw lifestyle work for me. After spending years using myself as a raw guinea pig, I finally figured out the aspects of the raw diet that work for me and which aspects that don't. I found that I thrive on raw organic vegetable and fruit juices and smoothies, probiotic-rich foods like kimchi and kombucha, fresh salads (when not flaring), nut milks, dehydrated raw cookies, crackers, and seaweeds. As I had only experienced mild flares since my 2010 hospitalization, I was finding that simple raw foods did, indeed, work out great for me. Gourmet raw foods are delicious to indulge in while not flaring, however, I save these as special treats only and do not have them incorporated into my everyday lifestyle because my colon has proved to me time and time again that gourmet raw foods do not work well with my system.

I started to miss warm and cooked foods, so the natural progression for me was to decide to completely go vegan. I enjoyed the vegan diet, felt empowered by not eating animals, but still, like on the raw diet, flared, though the flares were not nearly as severe and were controlled with a Hydrocortisone retention enema, which is Christmas compared to prednisone. While on the vegan diet, I ate mostly fruits and vegetables and avoided pre-packaged, highly processed, frozen, "shit" vegan foods that are only vegan by name and don't fulfill the intent of the vegan lifestyle. It was important to me to not be a "shit" vegan because that definitely would not be maximizing nutrients. Highly processed carbs and sugary vegan food would instead send naughty sugars right into my gut to feed the bad bacteria and, let me tell you, nothing good happens when bad bacteria completely takes over your gut! Sugar can call up the flare fairy for me, so I tried not to consume too much of it!

My vegan diet came to an abrupt end when I got pregnant with my first child. I distinctly remember waking up one morning and saying to my husband, "I want eggs and bacon, but I want the eggs cooked in the bacon grease!" I have never witnessed my husband jump out of bed faster than he did that morning. Talk about a drastic diet change! A few weeks earlier, I couldn't imagine eating bacon or eggs, let alone eggs cooked in bacon grease!! This was only a two-time occurrence during my first pregnancy, but it was good while it lasted!

During the duration of my pregnancy, I ate tons of kimchi and fermented foods. I simply could not get enough of these deliciously nutritious foods. I also couldn't get enough of hummus, pita, and Mediterranean soups. My other staple was Mexican food consisting of black bean tacos with onions and extra shredded cheese (yes, I started eating cheese again), or the infamous bean, cheese, rice, and onion burrito complete with chips and salsa from the local taqueria. Though these foods weren't on an everyday rotation. The foods that were on my normal rotation were lots of leafy greens, lots of fresh fruits and veggies, kombucha, beet kvass, and anything fresh and in season. I chose to eat mostly clean foods, but did not follow any traditional diet. I listened to my body and fed it (and my growing baby) accordingly. The only major aversion I had to any type of food during my first pregnancy was green juices and smoothies! For some reason, that particular nutritional elixir goodness was not welcome!

After giving birth to my daughter, I didn't follow any particular diet per se, but I did eat mostly whole foods, with the exception of my soy chai latte from Starbucks. That particular latte became my mommy indulgence, and my waistline quickly started showing it. I wanted to solely blame the prednisone that I had to take due to my post-partum flare for my rapid weight gain, but because I was nutritionally educated, I knew better. I repeated the mantra, *Fat doesn't make you fat. Sugar makes you fat!* But alas, I kept drinking it. Hey, I'm only human!

I was finally able to kick the Starbucks habit thanks to working with health coach extraordinaire Talia Pollock, and finally was able to completely turn my diet around! Though I was nutritionally educated, it's hard to hold yourself accountable. Like I said, I'm only human, so working with a health coach was key for me.

I became predominantly vegan and was eating plant based foods on a daily basis. Eating a whole foods diet and lifestyle dominated by fruits, veggies, nuts, seeds, and legumes was rocking my socks!

However, when I became pregnant in May of 2016, my love for the plant based lifestyle quickly died off again. The thought of smoothies and green juices repulsed me once again, and I didn't even have a taste for kimchi or any fermented type foods. All I wanted to eat was scrambled eggs, bread, pasta, cheese, and more bread and pasta! It was a win when I wanted pasta and green beans mixed together! Oh, yeah, and the occasional granny smith apple (thank God for that)! Though I didn't want to,

I forced myself to drink green juices blended with ice and avocado and would drink kombucha quite religiously, but other than that, I couldn't even look at a vegetable for the first trimester. I was part of a summer CSA and had planned to eat only off of the farm for the entire summer, but that definitely did not happen during the first trimester. I remember opening the fridge, packed with delicious, local, nutrient-dense organic produce and, instantly feeling repulsed, shut the fridge, thinking to myself, *What a travesty. I wish I could eat these veggies right now!* Luckily, as I entered my second trimester, my love for fruits, veggies, green juices and smoothies came back!

As I write this, I am currently four months pregnant and am enjoying eating mostly plants, but I still have an insatiable craving for organic eggs that I get from my local organic farmer. The main difference between my first and second pregnancies food wise is that I now love smoothies and green juices again, whereas, I was repulsed by these foods my entire first pregnancy.

My ultimate, overall goal is to strive to eat as nutritionally dense as possible. What I have learned from all of my "miracle diet" trials and errors is to create a meal plan that works for me and my unique needs. I have taken parts of each diet I have tried that worked for me and left the parts that didn't work behind. Through my trial and error, I was able to design my own bio-individual diet, meaning what works for me doesn't necessarily mean it will work for you, and vice-versa. Through this approach, I still have minor flares from time to time, but they are much milder than anything I experienced for the first four years after being diagnosed (minus my post-partum and pregnancy flares—those had a mind of their own).

I would never discourage another from trying a specific type of diet, including the fruitarian diet. I strongly feel that we each need to travel down our individual diet pathway, and by doing so, find what works for us and what doesn't. Some people respond immediately to *The Maker's Diet* or The Specific Carbohydrate Diet. To those that do, I tip my hat to you. To those of us that don't, there is hope; we just need to continue down the food trial and error pathway until we figure out what compliments our individual bodies best.

I have experienced countless frustrations when trying different diets, and have had more than my fair share of feeling like a failure because my body would not respond to several different "miracle" diets. In the end, I would not change a thing because this long and painstaking journey helped me realize that I am unique, my dietary needs are unique, and I am not a "one size fits all" person. I parallel diet to IBD drug treatment. No one person suffers exactly the same symptoms with their Crohn's or colitis, and there is not one blanket drug that works for everybody. The same is true for our individual dietary needs.

What I have found, after over ten years of trial and error, is that green juices and smoothies, organic meats, eggs, wild caught fish, bone broth, fermented foods and fermented beverages work best for me. Kombucha is almost a daily ritual for me! I try to avoid anything that is processed and comes from a box or can.

The occasional indulgences are always okay. We must all live a little! I'm a sucker for the occasional frozen margarita complete with a delicious Mexican dinner! The key is moderation and not very often.

Through this journey, I have learned that my disease truly does have a mind of its own. There were times I ate the cleanest diet on the planet, the raw foods diet, and still flared. There were times my daily diet consisted of a Starbucks venti soy chai tea latte and chips, salsa, and a bean-rice-onion-cheese burrito four times a week and thrived. When I think of that point in my life, I wonder if it was just sheer luck or the ultimate crap shoot. I'll never know. But I also know that way of eating is not the way our bodies were designed to optimally operate and thrive.

Find out what works for you, and remember, for ultimate health, eat clean, stress less, get plenty of rest, drink lots of water, and smile every day. Even if you're shitting your pants, keep smiling. I'm serious about that.

Take comfort in knowing that you will eventually figure out what works for you and your digestive tract. Be patient and love yourself, no matter how bleak things seem. Remember that eating clean, nutritious meals are important, but making sure that your mind, spirit, and soul are balanced and at peace are equally as important.

To you, I raise my green juice and say, *Kale Yeah! You can do this!!* Enjoy your food journey and make it your own based on your very unique and special bio-individual needs.

Let It Go

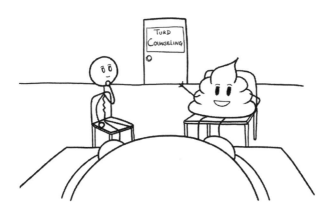

I can't believe it has been ten years since I came mano a mano with the bloody poo in my toilet. Nothing prepared me for that moment, and though it took a few months to figure out that I was going to have to live with the disease long-term, it took years for me to stop the all-out hand-to-hand combat that went on between me, my colon, and I.

I battled with inflammatory bowel disease for three and a half years before I lost my job because of my illness. Before losing my job, I literally forced myself to go to work every day, not allowing the disease to get the best of me. The people I worked for knew I was literally killing myself in the process and tried to get me to realize it, but I didn't. Call it the will of the human spirit, meat-headedness or just flat out denial, I'll never know. What I do know is that I realized how sick I truly was after being forced out of the Navy due to my diagnosis changing from ulcerative colitis to Crohn's disease. It was then that I found myself going through the painful process of explaining why I, at the ripe age of twenty-six, didn't have a job and couldn't actively search to get a new one due to the severity of my illness.

When I would meet somebody new at a gathering, dinner party, social function, you name it, I had to explain why I was not working. I felt that I had to explain to both acquaintances and complete strangers alike that though I looked perfectly healthy on the outside, that I was really sick on the inside. I had to deal with judgmental, ignorant assholes thinking that I was making this illness up because I *appeared* normal on the outside. What those assholes failed to realize was that World War III was going on in my gut, and had been for years. I didn't *appear* to be as ill as I really was simply because I was a tough cookie who refused to let the disease end my love for socializing, bike riding, and living my life. It amazed me how so-called rational, educated people couldn't wrap their minds around the concept that you can be extremely ill but continue living your life. They couldn't wrap their minds around the fact that I was extremely ill and couldn't control my bowels, but could still ride my bike. What they never knew was that I rode my bike hoping that I didn't crap myself in the process and prayed that my frail body could power me up even the smallest of hills. What they failed to realize is that I had to starve myself before attending any social function so I could guarantee that I wouldn't crap myself. I got tired of explaining. I got tired of the judgmental glances and snarky comments behind my back that others were making because I wasn't keeping up with the rat race. Finally, I grew some balls and decided to break it down "Barney style" for the judgmental masses, purple dinosaur and all.

It got to the point that if somebody asked me why I didn't work, I looked at them point blank and said, "I'm not working at the moment because I shit blood and, occasionally, myself." *Ha! Take that!* Their reaction? Priceless. Through that vivid description I provided to people, I started to gain my confidence back. Instead of feeling inadequate because I wasn't working, I started feeling inner strength and peace. I was slowly taking my life back. And that started with giving the finger to judgmental people who thought I was making up the severity and impact this disease had on my life. I was more than willing to tell somebody who thought I was making the disease up, "Hey, you're more than welcome to accompany me to the bathroom and I'll leave you something I guarantee you've NEVER seen before in the toilet." *Yeah, didn't think so.*

Having a disease that revolves around poo, bloody poo, 'rhea, and pooing yourself is not a proper dinner party topic. But it is reality. It happens. And if it is happening to you, accept it for what it is, grow strength from it, and learn to peacefully coexist with it. I literally spent seven years trying to conquer and eradicate colitis from my body, and in the process, was left frustrated with myself and banging my head against the wall wondering what I was doing wrong. I grew such hate and discontent towards my colon. *Why was this happening to me?* Why couldn't I have a normal, smooth colon versus an ulcerated, wound covered colon that felt and internally looked like I had crashed on my bike but somehow got the severe road rash inside my bowels, causing me to painfully shit blood.

I was tired of *always* looking in the toilet after I dropped a deuce to see if there was blood in my poo, and if so, how bad. I was tired of sprinting to the bathroom several times a day while flaring. If I was granted the blessing of remission, I was tired of constantly fearing the next flare. I was saddened that my once athletic, strong body was reduced to skin and bones when flaring, or fat and puffiness when put on prednisone to help get and keep me in remission. I just wanted to be normal, and greatly envied those who lived normal lives.

I became enraged when people would abuse their "normal" bodies with excessive alcohol consumption, recreational drugs, or junk foods. I cringed when people would brag about a drunken night of partying stupor. I became angry when people with healthy colons would complain about how bad their lives were. I became enraged when I saw people write "FML" on their Facebook feeds due to the pettiest of things. I found it incredulous that, in all these situations, they all took their "normal" colon and normal lives for granted. I wanted to shout at the top of my lungs, "NEWS FLASH! Your life is NOT that bad! You aren't dying! You aren't crapping your pants idiots! Stop being entitled morons!"

Due to being extremely ill, there were times that the darkness of depression took over my life. It happens to the best of us, even the most positive amongst us. I was so frustrated at times and couldn't understand why my entire body had to suffer the consequences of potent drugs to try and save the one piece of my body that didn't want to play well with others—my colon. I would get so angry because, though I would do absolutely *everything* right, I would still flare. I tried so many damn diets, ate as blandly as possibly, didn't drink anything but water and freshly juiced vegetables and fruit drinks, slept eight to ten hours a night, and my colon *still* flared. From initial diagnosis, I essentially let my entire life, and that of my husband's, revolve around my colon. I felt, at times, so damn powerless. I had no control of my colon, even after doing everything right.

These feelings bred bitterness and anger. There was a time in my life that I swore if my colon flared one more time, it was coming out. I began to despise my colon. I was done living my life around it. I felt that it had robbed me of my career, my self-confidence, my athletic ability, my health, and at times, my future. I felt left behind by the world. It seemed that everybody around me was progressing and I was somehow stuck in a stagnant cloud, not able to escape. I wanted to scream, and sometimes, I did. The bitterness, anger, fear, jealousy of the healthy among me, feelings of uncertainty and sadness about the present and future could only be expressed through breakdowns complete with screams and sobs. I just wanted to be normal! I wanted to be healthy! I DID NOT want to live my life around my sick colon! I did not want to have to worry when pre-planning a vacation if I would actually be healthy or flaring while on vacation. Dammit, I just wanted to live a normal, healthy, life!

When I would go into remission, I would set extremely lofty goals that would be unattainable even to the healthiest of beings. I decided that I was going to ride my bike and train intensely so I could be one of the top road cyclists in my area; maybe even become a pro cyclist—the sky was the limit, I thought! I wasn't shitting blood so I could do and accomplish anything I wanted, I thought. I had such lofty goals that, due to illness, I could never quite achieve because my body was not ready for such intense training and racing. But, as usual, I had to push the limits, only to fall short time after time. I tried for three years to defeat my illness by somehow ending up on the podium after a bike race. Unfortunately, that never happened.

After almost dying in 2010, I found solace, peace, and God in the mountains of Washington State. I also realized, for the first time, the biggest underlying struggle I possessed since being diagnosed in 2006.

I decided that I wanted to summit Mount Rainier for my 30th birthday and summit Mount Everest for my 40th. I planned on setting up a fundraising page titled "Emma to Everest" to help collect donations. I was hoping that my inspirational story would rally the masses to help me fund such an expensive, challenging goal. I felt that if I could achieve the difficult task of summiting Everest then my disease would not own me and would not dictate what my life would be like.

My husband, recognizing what was going on, told me to take it one step at a time, but knew deep down that my stubborn nature was yet again taking me to the extreme, like it had with my cycling goals. He did not want me to go through the same vicious cycle with mountaineering. It wasn't until we were at dinner with our close friends that the inconvenient truth came to light. After explaining to my close friends my summit goals, they knew the true driving force behind it. They saw me fall short with my cycling goals, not because I didn't try hard enough or because I wasn't capable of reaching them had I been healthy, but because the illness was a bit too much for my body to handle at the time. Directly put, my friend looked at me and said, "Achieving the impossible is not going to make you happy."

I began to cry as a great realization released itself from the depths of my inner being. At that moment, it all made sense. Since being diagnosed in 2006, I had pushed myself, to a fault, to achieve things that were far-fetched in the hopes that I could prove to myself that ulcerative colitis did not run my life. I felt that if I could win a bike race or summit numerous mountains that I would validate myself as an individual. What I failed to realize was that those who matter most to me do not care about any of those things. They just want me to be happy, healthy and to not waste time chasing "dreams" fueled by misguided emotions. Achieving what most never do, such as summiting Everest or becoming a pro cyclist, would not change my shitty circumstances. Achieving what seems like the impossible would not change my diagnosis. It would not heal my colon. Only I could do that—not things or events that I attained. It was then that I began to truly shift my mindset.

Though I became super frustrated at times, I never lost hope. Through years of prednisone usage, intravenous biologic treatment, medicine-driven extreme weight gain and sickness-induced severe weight loss, repeated failures to achieve unattainable goals, flare after flare, I never lost faith and hope. I always believed that I would heal, even while being succumbed by the darkness of depression. To this day, I do believe that I will fully heal. I do believe that I will live medicine-free. I believe that I will one day not have a suppressed immune system. The only difference now is that I no longer fight my disease. My primary goal is not to eradicate colitis from my body, but to coexist peacefully with it.

Inflammatory bowel disease has taught me so much about life. It has taught me to let go of ego, pride, and things that don't matter. It has taught me that my health comes first, because without health, we have nothing. It has taught me that a strong, loving, supporting relationship with family and friends is necessary. It has taught me that I can literally shit my pants, be knocking on death's door, and still live to tell about it. It has taught me that I am not defined by anything other than what I possess in my soul. It has taught me that though I suffer from it, I am not defined by it.

I want to remind you that you are not defined by your disease, you are simply unique because of it. I spent many months while flaring beating my head against the wall wondering what it would be like if I didn't have this illness. I wondered what it would be like to be normal. I wished that I didn't always look in the toilet after I crapped to ensure there wasn't any blood in my poo. I wished I didn't have to be on prednisone and blow up like a blimp. I wished I didn't display such anger and rage towards those closest to me while on prednisone. I wished I could have a healthy body and be medicine-free. I wished I could be normal.

That was all then. There is no point in wondering "what if" or wishing you didn't have the disease. Accept your illness for what it is, make peace with it, try and find the positives, leave the negatives, take a deep breath, and let it go. Try and move on with your life!

To those suffering right alongside me, I want to tell you that your life is beautiful, has so much meaning, and is so full of promise. And believe it or not, your digestive tract is beautiful too. It is telling you to change your life for the better and to start paying attention to your body. I neglected mine for years, and my colon revolted, changing my entire way of life, ultimately for the better.

Don't let flare after flare knock your spirit down and keep your morale in the toilet. If you are put on a potent medication to help heal your digestive tract, remember that it is needed at the moment to help you heal, and you can use it as a tool to help you get healthy and vibrant once again. Once healthy and vibrant, you may be able to come off of it. Never lose hope on that.

If you shit your pants, know that you aren't alone; the best among us have all done it, so don't dwell, just let it go. If you have to drive around with a makeshift toilet, accept it for what it is, acknowledge that it is temporary, and let it go. If a person you are dating is grossed out by your disease, first tell them to go pound sand because they're not worth your time, and let them go without looking back. If you don't jive with your doctor, fire them, and find another doc that you do work well with. All docs aren't created equal, and when you find the right one, you'll know.

There were times I never thought I would go into long-term remission, and times I almost died due to the disease. I accepted those situations for what they were, tried to find the lesson and the beauty in each, and let them go. I am still on my healing journey and still hope to one day be completely healed and medicine-free.

The best advice I can give is this: Learn to peacefully coexist with your disease, find the positives in it, and let the embarrassing shit go. Literally.

93012592R00062

Made in the USA
San Bernardino, CA
06 November 2018